Atlas of
MR Pathology

Deborah L. Durham, BS, RT(R) (MR) (CT)

Forsyth Technical Community College
Winston-Salem, North Carolina

W.B. SAUNDERS COMPANY
A Division of Harcourt Brace & Company

Philadelphia ■ London ■ Toronto ■ Montreal ■ Sydney ■ Tokyo

W.B. SAUNDERS COMPANY
A Division of Harcourt Brace & Company

The Curtis Center
Independence Square West
Philadelphia, Pennsylvania 19106

Library of Congress Cataloging-in-Publication Data

Durham, Deborah L.
Atlas of MR pathology / Deborah L. Durham.

p.   cm.

ISBN 0–7216–6416–4

1. Magnetic resonance imaging—Atlases.   I. Title.
[DNLM: 1. Head—radiography—atlases.   2. Neck—radiography—atlases.
3. Spine—radiography—atlases.   4. Musculoskeletal System—
radiography—atlases.   WE 17 D961a 1997]

RC78.7.N83D87 1997   616.07′548—dc20

DNLM/DLC   96–8867

ATLAS OF MR PATHOLOGY   ISBN 0–7216–6416–4

Printed in the United States of America.

Last digit is the print number: 9   8   7   6   5   4   3   2   1

To Leesa, Kiltie, Emmy, and Jordie—
who taught me to live, love, and survive

Preface

The most important goal of this atlas is to provide a coffee table book–like, fun approach for MR technologists and students to learn about the disease processes they are helping to diagnose. Images included are the "real" thing, not "doctored" as in so many other texts.

A brief overview of MR technology is given to help in understanding the pathologies seen using a variety of MR imaging techniques. Reference tables are in Chapter 1 to assist with review of the pathology charts for each disease process.

The atlas chapters were determined according to the specifications given by the American Registry of Radiologic Technologists for their national examination on magnetic resonance imaging. This volume can thereby be used as a learning and teaching tool for this examination.

Acknowledgments

I wish to thank and acknowledge all those who were instrumental in the preparation of this atlas.

I am especially grateful to John Briggs for all of the photography of the scans. He did a tremendous job.

Thanks to Sherri Poore for helping with the computer and the word processing of the manuscript.

A special thanks to the MR technologists at Forsyth Memorial Hospital in Winston-Salem, North Carolina, and the MR technologists at North Carolina Baptist Hospital, especially Gay Luebchow, for assisting me in gathering some of the pathology examples from their institute.

Thanks to the MR technologists at High Point Regional Hospital in High Point, North Carolina—Carol, Debbe, Amy, and Teresa—first of all, for being my friends, and, second, for always allowing me to look over their shoulders.

I want to thank Dave Zaritsky, MD, and William Woodruff, MD, for all of their help in answering my endless questions. Thanks to "Z" for always making me laugh and look at my potential.

A special thanks to James Sanderford, MD, for being my medical advisor for this atlas and for giving me needed counsel.

I am very grateful to my present and previous students for all their questions. These students were the inspiration for this atlas—to help them learn more about the different disease processes. This volume, it is hoped, will benefit students in all of the health-related technologies.

I am most grateful to all my friends and fellow faculty members and to my dean for their encouragement and support for this project.

A simple thank you to Jim and Luli for all they have done for the past 18 years.

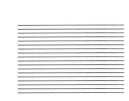

Contents

CHAPTER ONE

Reference Review

Magnetic resonance imaging is a complicated technology with numerous manufacturers and their various terms. A simple overview of MR concepts is given to provide a better understanding of the diseases in this book.

MRI involves the use of magnetic fields, radiofrequency fields, and hydrogen protons, which possess magnetic characteristics. Hydrogen protons make up 80% of the human body and allow signals to be received from them to create textbook-like images. The main static magnetic fields' strength is measured in tesla (T) units. Clinical MR systems are usually from .5 T to 1.5 T. The diseases discussed in this book were scanned on 1.5-T units. This should be kept in mind when reviewing suggested scan parameters. Also needed for MR imaging is a radiofrequency generator to create a radiofrequency field to excite the hydrogen protons in the body, and yet another set of magnetic fields are generated to allow specific slices in specific anatomic planes to be imaged.

Whenever the patient is placed into the scanner (area of interest is in the center of the main field) (Fig. 1–1), a net magnetization of the body occurs because a majority of the hydrogen protons align with the main magnetic field. Depending on the strength of the main magnetic field, the hydrogen protons spin at a specific rate. (At 1.5 T the hydrogen protons precess at around 63 MH.) The radiofrequency field is set

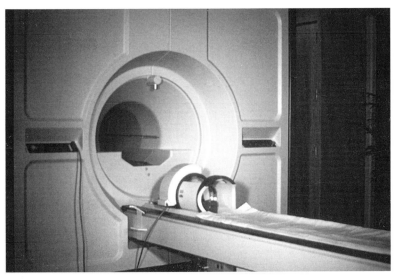

Figure 1–1 1.5 T magnet

to match this frequency or this rate to excite the hydrogen protons and change the net magnetization into a plane that is 90 degrees away from the original plane. If the net magnetization of the patient is originally in the Z plane (longitudinal), then the net magnetization is moved into the XY plane. This is the usual configuration of the 1.5-T clinical MR systems. In order for a signal to be received from the hydrogen protons, the net magnetization must be in the XY plane. Good images require good signals. As you can see, it is very important for the radiofrequency field (pulse) to match the precessing hydrogen protons. When the radiofrequency pulse is turned off, the hydrogen protons return to their original position in the longitudinal plane. This return to origination is termed *relaxation.*

There are two main types of relaxation: T1 and T2. T1 is the return of the net magnetization into the longitudinal plane. T2 is the decay of the net magnetization in the XY plane. T1 and T2 certainly sound like the same thing, but they are two completely different processes. T1 and T2 imaging sequences are examined later in this chapter.

First, we need to identify how the gradient magnetic fields fit in the picture. They allow for specific slices in certain anatomic planes to be imaged. Coils of wire along the sides of the bore of the magnet are switched on and off by electricity, thereby creating an additional magnetic field imposed on the main static magnetic field. This is done at specific times to create different rates of spin of the hydrogen protons. Remember: the frequency of the spin of the hydrogen protons must be matched by the radiofrequency field. All of this allows for different slices of the body to be scanned in different anatomic planes. The gradient fields can also be used to help generate the actual signals back from the body.

T1 and T2 relaxations and their time variances are used to create imaging sequences. All relaxation times are based on fat and water. This is where most of the body's hydrogen protons are found. Whenever T1 relaxation of a tissue needs to be studied, a T1-weighted scan sequence is performed. T1 images are known for their anatomic detail. Fat appears white, and fluid, such as cerebrospinal fluid, appears black or dark. When T2 relaxation needs to be studied, T2-weighted images are done, in which fat appears gray and fluid appears white. T2-weighted images are known for their contrast. Proton density images are a combination of the two. These types of images specifically look at the concentration of hydrogen protons in the slice. To achieve T1- and T2-weighted images, certain scan parameters are manipulated. Scan sequences are created using parameters involving timing of the excitation radiofrequency pulse and listening to (receiving) the signal back from a slice of tissue (Tables 1–1, 1–2).

Magnetic Resonance Angiogram

Obviously, there are many varied sequences to create innumerable MR images. MR angiogram sequences are manipulated to look at flowing blood in the body. The most common sequence uses the time of flight theory. Time of flight looks at the differences between blood flowing into a slice and the stationary tissue in the slice. This allows for the blood to appear bright against darkened background tissue. The slices scanned by this technique are then postprocessed to create an "arteriogram-like" image (Fig. 1–2).

Surface Coils

An important part of MR imaging in diagnosing disease processes is the correct selection of a surface coil to match the body part being examined. A surface coil is

Table 1–1. **Parameter Chart**

Parameter	Description
Echo time (TE)	When the signal is taken from the tissues
Repetition time (TR)	Time from one excitation RF pulse to the next excitation RF pulse for one slice
Flip angle	How far the net magnetization is transferred into the XY plane
Matrix	Phase encodes and frequency encodes to fill up computer data space to create the image; number of phase encodes affects scan time
Acquisition (average)	The number of times a tissue is sampled
Slice thickness	The thickness of the slice that is scanned
Slice gap	Distance between slices
Field of view	Area of interest
Echo train length	Number of echoes listened to before next excitation pulse; affects phase encodes and scan time
Magnet strength	1.5 T

RF = radiofrequency.

placed around, below, or on top of the body part being imaged to highlight the area. The field of view can also be reduced according to coil limitations to create an even better detailed image. The surface coils can transmit the radiofrequency field needed for a sequence or receive the signal back from the tissue. Some coils, such as the head coil, can do both. Surface coils will vary, depending on the manufacturer. It is suggested that technologists follow vendor specifications with regard to the use of the surface coils (Table 1–3).

Contrast

In 1989, the U.S. Food and Drug Administration approved an intravenous contrast agent for use with MR imaging. The contrast used for MR is a gadolinium chelate, a paramagnetic compound that changes the local magnetic fields of the tissue through

Text continued on page 9

Table 1–2. **Sequence Chart**

Variable	Sequence
T1 weighted	Short TE, short TR
T2 weighted	Long TE, long TR
Proton density	Short TE, long TR
Gradient echo T1 weighted	Greater than 45-degree flip angle, short TE, short TR
Gradient echo T2 weighted	Less than 45-degree flip angle, short TE, short TR
Magnetic resonance angiography	Time of flight technique with short TE, short TR

TE = echo time; TR = repetition time.

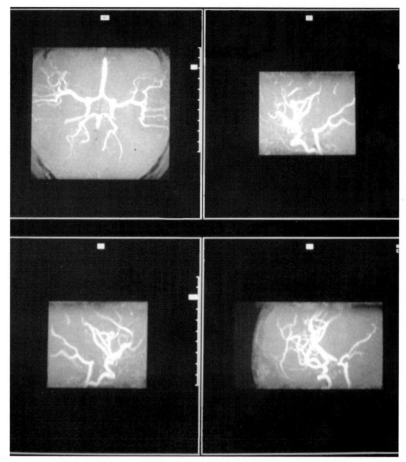

Figure 1-2 Example of MRA

Table 1-3. **Examples of Surface Coils**

Body Part	Surface Coil
Head	Head, face, feet, ankles (Fig. 1–3) MRA: circle of Willis, carotids
Extremity	Shoulder (Fig. 1–4) Knee (Fig. 1–5)
Small field of view	Wrist (Fig. 1–6) Temporomandibular joint (Fig. 1–7)
Spine	Thoracic, lumbar (Fig. 1–8)
Neck	Cervical, neck (Fig. 1–9)
Endorectal coil (placed inside rectum before scanning)	Rectum, bladder, prostate, uterus

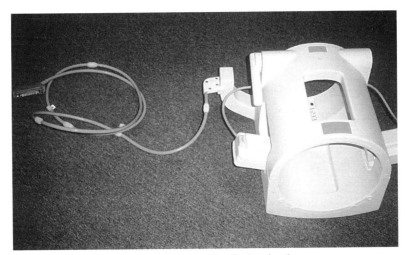

Figure 1–3 Example of a head coil

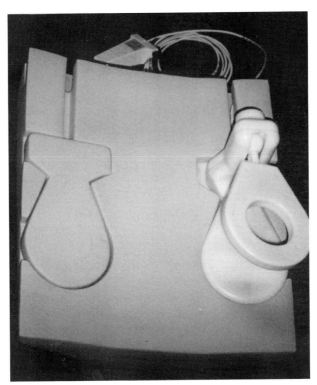

Figure 1–4 Example of a shoulder coil

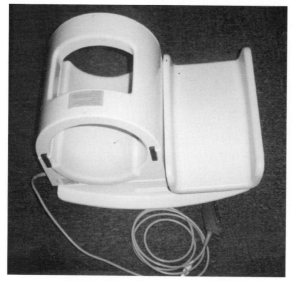

Figure 1-5 Example of a knee coil

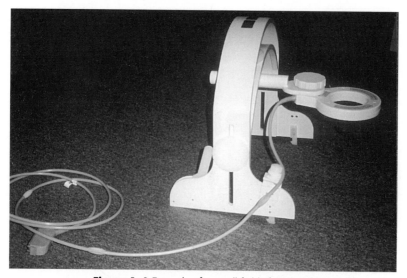

Figure 1-6 Example of a small field-of-view coil

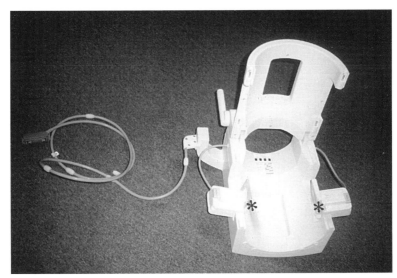

Figure 1-7 Example of a temporomandibular joint coil

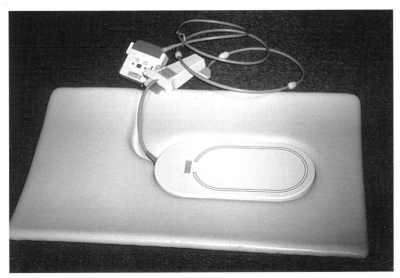

Figure 1-8 Example of a spine coil

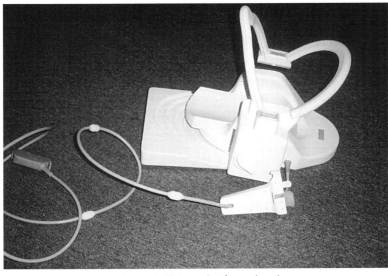

Figure 1-9 Example of a neck coil

Table 1–4. **Common Protocols**

Routine head	T1 sagittal: 7 mm
	T2 axial: 5–6 mm
	T1 axial-coronal: 5 mm
	FOV = 220–230 mm
	Matrix = 256 × 256/192 × 256
Routine cervical spine	T1 sagittal: 4 mm
	T2 sagittal: 4 mm
	T2 axial: 4 mm
	FOV = 280 mm
	Matrix = 192 × 256
Routine thoracic spine	T1 sagittal: 5 mm
	T1 sagittal: 5 mm
	T2 sagittal: 5 mm
	T2 axial if needed
	FOV = 500 mm (body sequence) or 300 mm (thoracic)
	Matrix = 192 × 256
Routine lumbar spine	T1 sagittal: 5 mm
	T2 sagittal: 5 mm
	T2 axial: 5 mm
	FOV = 280 mm
	Matrix = 192 × 256
Routine shoulder	T1 paracoronal: 4 mm
	T2 paracoronal: 4 mm
	T2 axials: 4 mm
	T1 parasagittals: 4 mm
	FOV = 180 mm
	Matrix = 256 × 256
Routine knee	T1 sagittal: 4 mm
	T2 sagittal: 4 mm
	T2 coronal: 4 mm
	Axials if previous surgery
	FOV = 160 mm
	Matrix = 192 × 256
Routine temporomandibular joint	T1 sagittals: both sides
	Gradient echo T2 single slice with ratchet to show opening movement of jaw
	FOV = 130 mm
	Matrix = 256 × 256
Routine hips	T1 coronal: 6 mm
	T2 coronal: 6 mm
	T1 axials: 6 mm
	T2 axials: 6 mm (if fracture suspected)
	FOV = 400 mm
	Matrix = 256 × 256
Routine soft tissue neck	T1 sagittal: 4–5 mm
	T2 sagittal: 4–5 mm
	T1 axials: 4–5 mm
	T2 axials: 4–5 mm
	FOV = 250 mm
	Matrix = 192 × 256
Routine MR angiography of the brain	Three-dimensional gradient echo T2 axial (TR = 29 ms, TE = 7 ms, flip angle = 20)
	80-mm slab with saturation area above
	Postprocessing of raw scan data for arteriogram-like images
Routine MR angiography of the carotids	Two-dimensional gradient echo T2
	54 slices at 4 mm
	Three-dimensional gradient echo T2
	Slab of 64 mm
	Postprocessing of raw scan data for arteriogram-like images
Angiography of the heart	T1 axials
	T1 paracoronal
	T2 paracoronal
	ECG triggered
	FOV = 400

FOV = field of view; TR = repetition time; TE = echo time; ECG = electrocardiogram.

which it traverses. Three drug companies now produce different variations of this compound. The gadolinium serves the same purpose as the x-ray dye in that it enhances tumors, infections, and certain disease processes. Common dosage is from 10 to 20 mL, depending on patient weight. T1-weighted sequences are used after contrast injection.

Summary

With the brief discussion of the interaction of the magnetic fields and hydrogen protons in the body along with parameter and sequence charts (Table 1–4), the images in this book should provide a good learning tool for MR diseases.

CHAPTER TWO

Head and Neck

Chart 2–1. **Head and Neck** (Fig. 2–1)

Pathology	Arachnoid cyst
Description	Cerebrospinal fluid–filled pocket located between the dura and pia mater layers of the meninges; could develop as a result of adhesions from infection or trauma
Symptoms	Asymptomatic unless cyst pressing on vital structure
Suggested protocols	Routine head
Appearance	Dark on T1 White on T2 Should not enhance
Contrast	To differentiate from other lesions

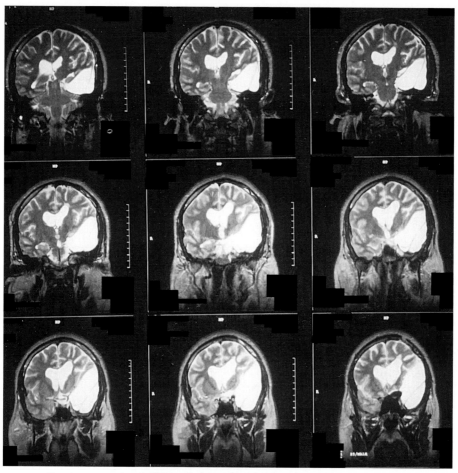

Figure 2-1 Arachnoid cyst
T2-weighted coronals

Chart 2–2. **Head and Neck** (Figs. 2–2 and 2–3)

Pathology	Subdural hematoma
Description	Collection of blood between the dura and subarachnoid spaces as a result of the rupture of veins that bridge the venous system of brain to the intradural venous sinuses; acute subdurals are due to trauma; chronic subdurals can grow slowly in older people and alcoholics
Symptoms	Headaches, confusion, fluctuating levels of consciousness, bruise or injury to one side of the head
Suggested protocols	Routine head
Appearance	White on all T2 images Lighter in signal on T1 images
Contrast	Does not enhance with contrast

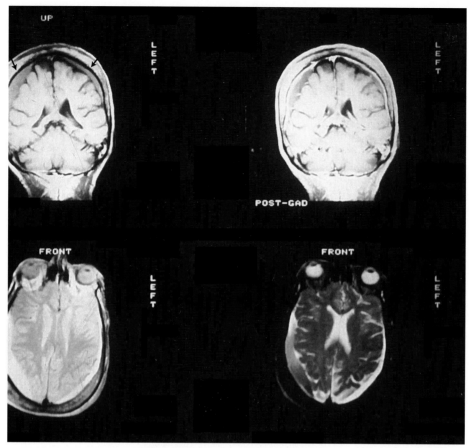

Figure 2-2 Bilateral subdural hematoma
Upper right: T1 coronal after contrast
Upper left: T1 coronal before contrast
Lower left: proton density axial
Lower right: T2 axial

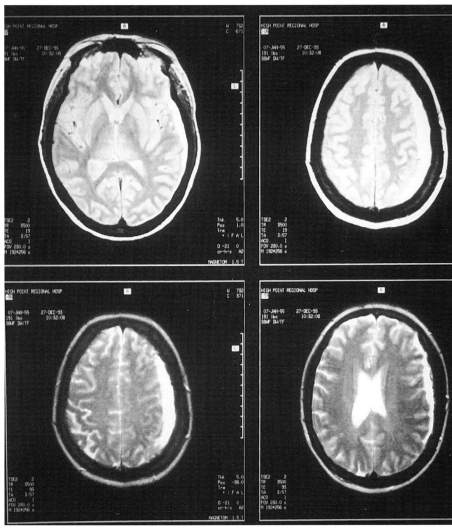

Figure 2–3 Left subdural hematoma
Upper left: proton density axial
Upper right: proton density axial
Lower left: T2 axial
Lower right: T2 axial

Chart 2–3. **Head and Neck** (Figs. 2–4 and 2–5)

Pathology	Hydrocephalus
Description	Increased abnormal volume of cerebrospinal fluid, which causes an enlargement of the ventricular system in the brain; occurs because of a blockage in the ventricular system, which could result from congenital malformations, infections, subarachnoid hemorrhage, and lesions pushing on the ventricular system
Symptoms	Dementia, gait disturbance, headache, nausea, papilledema (edema of the optic disc)
Suggested protocols	Routine head with or without contrast
Appearance	Enlarged black ventricles on T1 Enlarged white ventricles on T2
Contrast	May be necessary to highlight a lesion invading the ventricular system causing a blockage

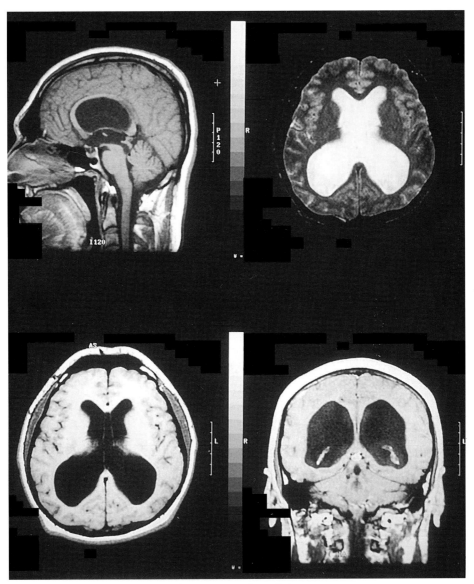

Figure 2–4 Hydrocephalus
Upper left: T1 sagittal
Upper right: T2 axial
Lower left: T1 axial
Lower right: T1 coronal

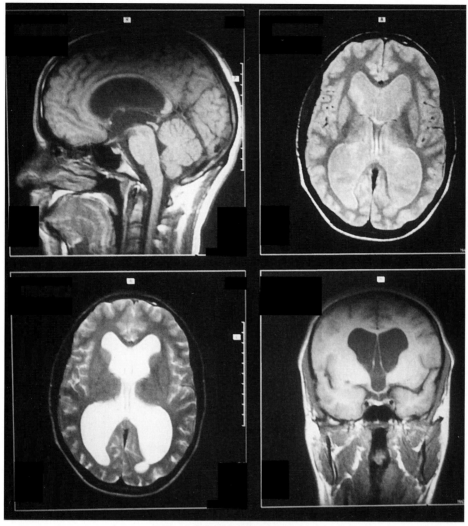

Figure 2–5 Hydrocephalus
Upper left: T1 sagittal
Upper right: proton density axial
Lower left: T2 axial
Lower right: T1 coronal

Chart 2–4. **Head and Neck** (Fig. 2–6)

Pathology	Cerebellopontine angle lesion
Description	Intra-axial lesion that arises at the angle of junction between the cerebellum and the pons
Symptoms	Dizziness or hearing loss because of close proximity to seventh and eighth cranial nerves
Suggested protocols	Routine brain with contrast Thin slices through internal auditory canals and pons Pre- and postcontrast (axial-coronal)
Appearance	Not well visualized on T1 Area of edema (white) around pons and internal auditory canals
Contrast	To show boundaries of lesion

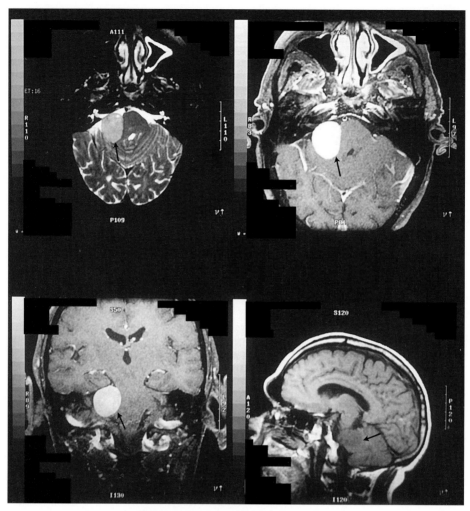

Figure 2–6 Cerebellopontine angle lesion
Upper left: T2 axial
Upper right: T1 axial (contrast)
Lower left: T1 coronal (contrast)
Lower right: T1 sagittal

Chart 2–5. **Head and Neck** (Figs. 2–7 and 2–8)

Pathology	Pituitary gland tumor (Fig. 2–7) Hypervascular adenoma (Fig. 2–8)
Description	Mass arising from the anterior or posterior lobe of the pituitary gland (varying in size) occurs in persons 20 to 50 years old; classified as microadenoma (<1 cm) or macroadenoma (>1 cm)
Symptoms	Blurred vision Menstrual irregularities Increased prolactin levels in blood
Suggested protocols	Coronal and sagittal before and after contrast 3-mm slices FOV = 200
Appearance	Enlarged sella turcica on T1 Contrast differences between mass and gland on T2
Contrast	Tumors could appear dark immediately after contrast Tumors could appear bright 20 to 30 minutes after contrast Hypervascular adenomas are bright throughout

FOV = field of view.

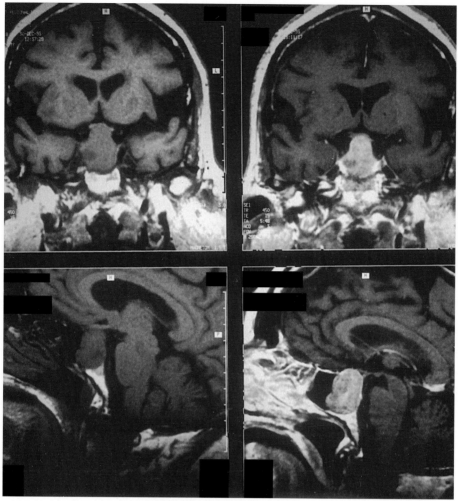

Figure 2–7 Pituitary gland lesion
Upper left: T1 coronal
Upper right: T1 coronal (contrast)
Lower left: T1 sagittal
Lower right: T1 sagittal (contrast)

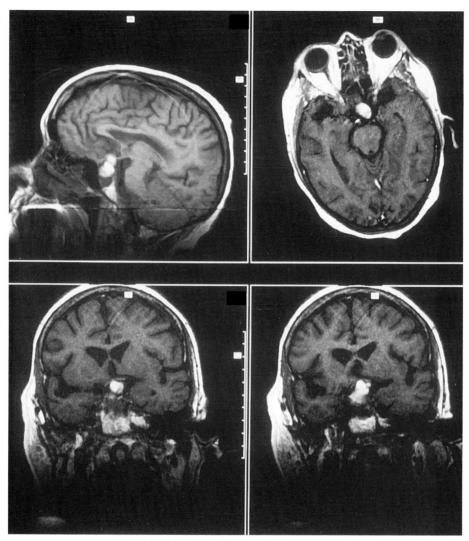

Figure 2–8 Hypervascular adenoma of the pituitary gland
Upper left: T1 sagittal
Upper right: T1 axial
Lower left: T1 coronal
Lower right: T1 coronal

Chart 2–6. **Head and Neck** (Figs. 2–9 and 2–10)

Pathology	Metastases to brain
Description	Lesions that arise from cancer cells that have traveled to the gray-white matter junctions in the brain
Symptoms	Seizures, headaches, blurry vision, or various neurologic symptoms
Suggested protocols	Routine head All three planes after contrast for possible surgical intervention
Appearance	Areas of edema: white on T2 images, dark on T1 images
Contrast	Needed for enhancement of actual lesion versus edema

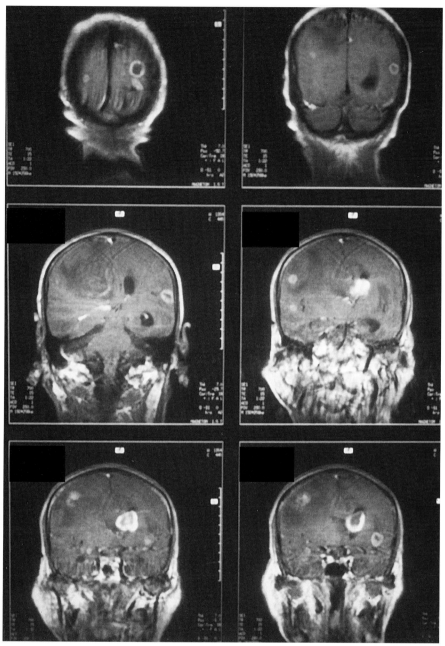

Figure 2–9 Metastases to the brain
T1 coronals (contrast)

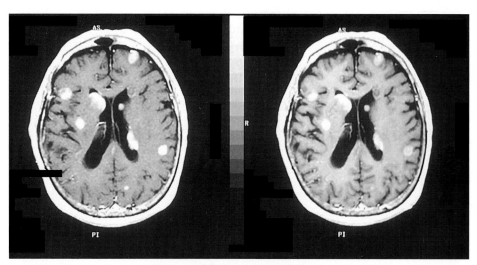

Figure 2-10 Metastases to the brain
T1 axials (contrast)

Chart 2–7. **Head and Neck** (Fig. 2–11)

Pathology	Acoustic neuroma
Description	Extra-axial lesion arising from the eighth (vestibulocochlear) cranial nerve, usually benign
Symptoms	Hearing loss on affected side Dizziness
Suggested protocols	Routine brain Thin sections through internal auditory canals, axial and coronal (after contrast)
Appearance	Without contrast: widening of internal auditory canal With contrast: bright, allowing delineation of boundaries of lesion
Contrast	To visualize lesion borders

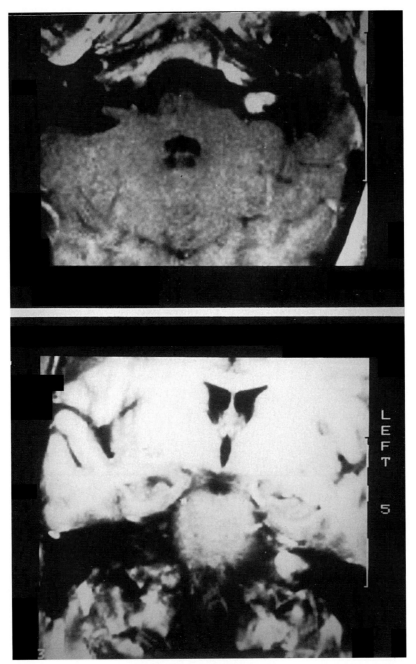

Figure 2-11 Acoustic neuroma
Upper: T1 axial (contrast)
Lower: T1 coronal (contrast)

Chart 2–8. **Head and Neck** (Figs. 2–12 and 2–13)

Pathology	Pineal gland lesion (see Fig. 2–12) Pineal gland cyst or lesion (see Fig. 2–13)
Description	Lesion could be benign or a low-grade malignancy; occurs mainly in adults; cysts are fluid filled
Symptoms	Depending on size of lesion, could cause pressure on ventricular system, headaches, and other neurologic variances
Suggested protocols	Routine brain with contrast
Appearance	Cyst: dark on T1, white on T2 Lesion will have edema (white) on T2 Abnormal signal on T1
Contrast	To differentiate solid versus cystic components

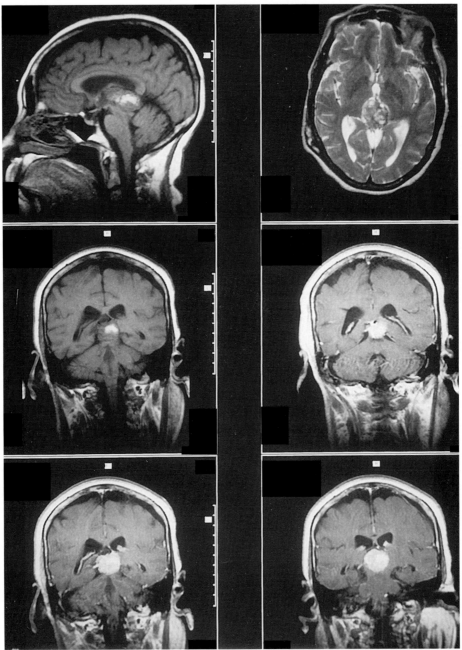

Figure 2-12 Pineal gland lesion
Upper left: T1 sagittal (contrast)
Upper right: T2 axial
Middle left: T1 coronal (contrast)
Middle right: T1 coronal (contrast)
Lower left: T1 coronal (contrast)
Lower right: T1 coronal (contrast)

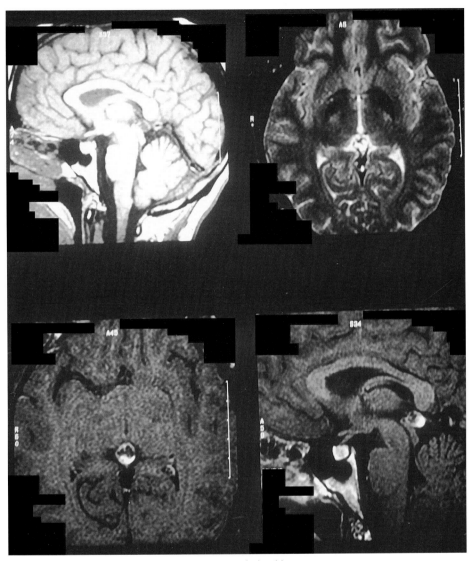

Figure 2–13 Pineal gland lesion or cyst
Upper left: T1 sagittal
Upper right: T2 axial
Lower left: T1 axial (contrast)
Lower right: T1 sagittal (contrast)

Chart 2-9. **Head and Neck** (Figs. 2-14 to 2-16)

Pathology	Optic glioma
Description	Rare neoplasm of optic nerve; low-grade tumor that grows slowly over several years; occurs in children
Symptoms	Vision problems Headaches
Suggested protocols	Routine brain with contrast All three planes after contrast
Appearance	Edema (white) on T2 Edema (dark) on T1 Bright with contrast
Contrast	Enhances well to visualize borders and invasiveness

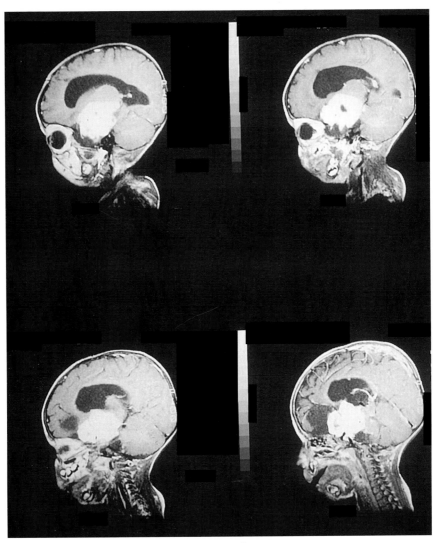

Figure 2-14 Optic glioma
T1 sagittals (contrast)

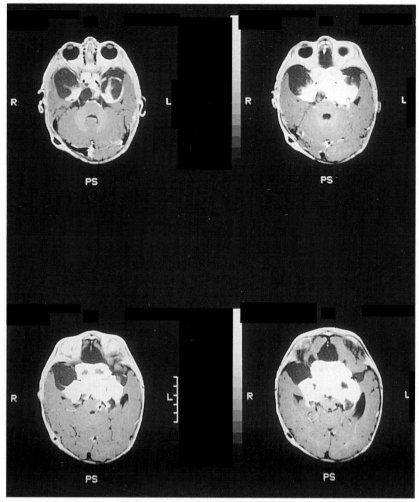

Figure 2–15 Optic glioma
T1 axials (contrast)

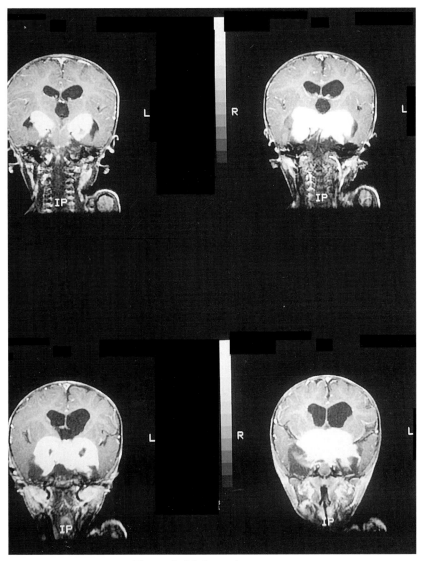

Figure 2–16 Optic glioma
T1 coronals (contrast)

Chart 2–10. **Head and Neck** (Fig. 2–17)

Pathology	Recurrent optic nerve melanoma on right Left eye removed
Description	Occurs almost exclusively in white adults; elevated pigmented nodule in optic nerve grows rapidly, metastases through lymph and blood
Symptoms	Vision problems Optic neuritis
Suggested protocols	Routine brain Thin cuts at the angle of the optic nerve A fat saturation scan sequence to void out all fat in area to visualize globe, muscles, and nerve
Appearance	Irregularity of optic nerve Difficult to see edema around nerve unless lesion has invaded other surrounding tissues
Contrast	Enhancement of lesion

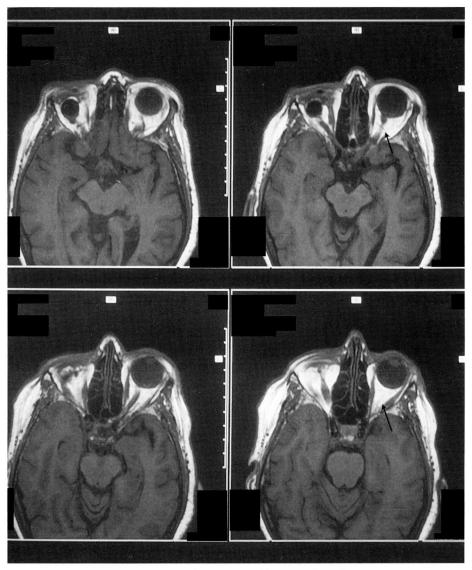

Figure 2-17 Left eye, removed because of a melanoma
Right eye, recurrent melanoma
Upper left: T1 axial
Upper right: T1 axial
Lower left: T1 axial
Lower right: T1 axial (contrast)

Chart 2–11. **Head and Neck** (Fig. 2–18)

Pathology	Cholesteatoma
Description	Squamous epithelium forms a pearly white mass from acute and chronic inflammation; occurs from chronic otitis media; forms usually in the middle ear
Symptoms	Imbalance Earache Dizziness Hearing loss on affected side
Suggested protocols	Routine brain Thin cuts through internal auditory canals and petrous area
Appearance	White on T2 around petrous area Dark on T1 around petrous area
Contrast	To enhance acute infectious process

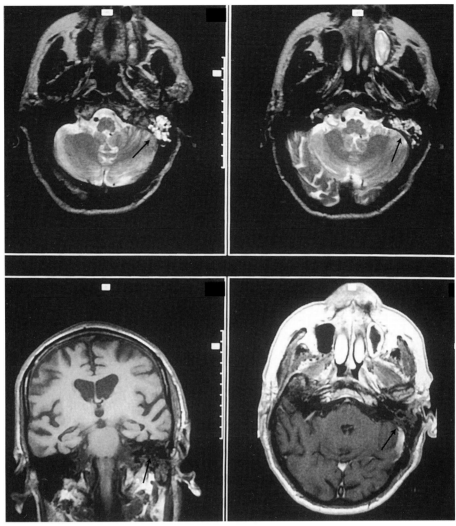

Figure 2–18 Cholesteatoma
Upper left: T2 axial
Upper right: T2 axial
Lower left: T1 coronal
Lower right: T1 axial

Chart 2–12. **Head and Neck** (Fig. 2–19)

Pathology	Maxillofacial lesion
Description	Could be a metastasis or a primary cancer
Symptoms	Sinus stuffiness Fullness in face Pain
Suggested protocols	Routine head with centering to include all of facial bones
Appearance	Asymmetric facial soft tissues Gray signal from soft tissue lesion instead of black as normal maxillary sinuses appear
Contrast	To evaluate extent and boundaries of lesion

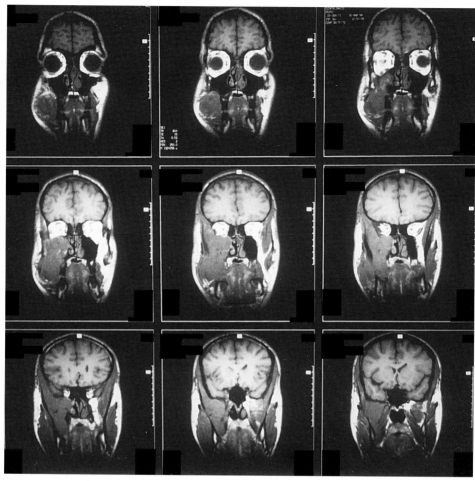

Figure 2–19 Maxillofacial lesion, left side involving sinuses and orbit
T1 coronals

Chart 2–13. **Head and Neck** (Figs. 2–20 to 2–22)

Pathology	Multiple sclerosis
Description	Demyelinating disease; presence of plaques of demyelination in the white matter, usually around optic nerve and paraventricular regions; occurs mostly in women 20 to 50 years old
Symptoms	Vision problems: optic neuritis Weakness Tingling in extremities
Suggested protocols	Routine brain with contrast
Appearance	Bright "flame"-shaped areas in white matter on T2 Not well visualized on T1
Contrast	Active plaques enhance

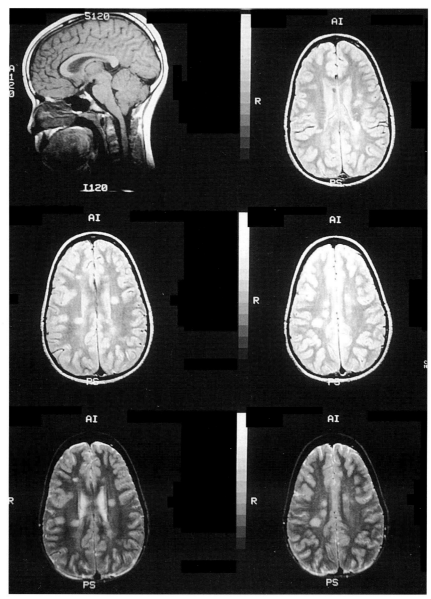

Figure 2–20 Multiple sclerosis
Upper left: T1 sagittal
Upper right: proton density axial
Middle: proton density axials
Lower: T2 axials

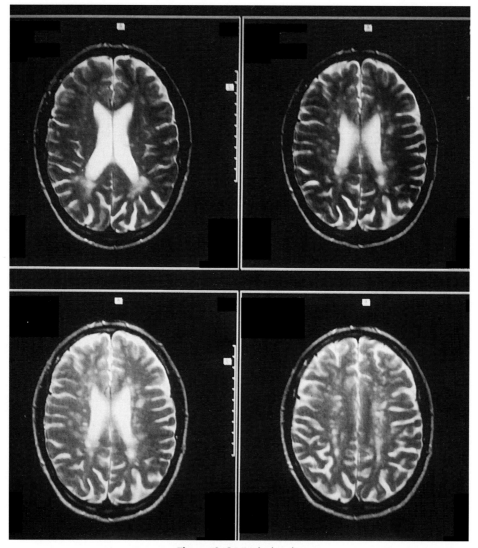

Figure 2–21 Multiple sclerosis
Upper: T2 axials
Lower: T2 axials

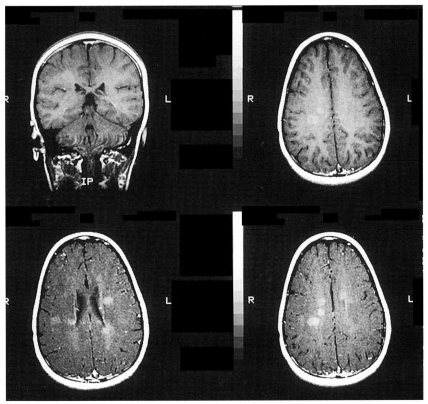

Figure 2–22 Multiple sclerosis
Upper left: T1 coronal (contrast)
Upper right: T1 axial (contrast)
Lower left: T1 axial (contrast)
Lower right: T1 axial (contrast)

Chart 2–14. **Head and Neck** (Fig. 2–23)

Pathology	Cerebellar infarct (stroke)
Description	Area of necrotic cells surrounded by edema caused by a thrombus or an embolus to vertebrobasilar system
Symptoms	Tremors, incoordination, hypotonia
Suggested protocols	Routine brain Thin sections through cerebellum
Appearance	Edema (white) in cerebellum on T2 Edema (dark) in cerebellum on T1
Contrast	Could be used to differentiate from lesion

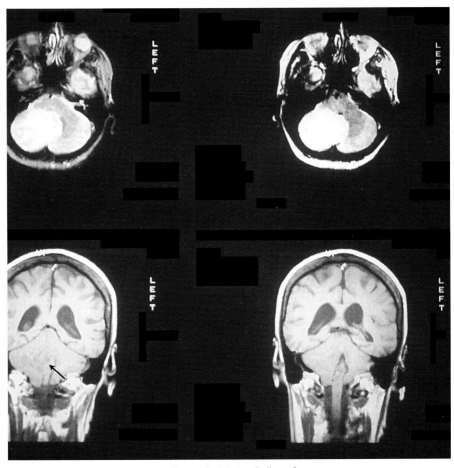

Figure 2–23 Cerebellar infarct
Upper: T2 axials
Lower: T1 coronals

Chart 2–15. **Head and Neck** (Figs. 2–24 and 2–25)

Pathology	Midbrain infarct (stroke)
Description	Necrosis of brain tissue in area secondary to vessel occlusion
Symptoms	Vision problems, motor function difficulties
Suggested protocols	Routine brain with contrast Axial and coronal through brain stem 3–4 mm
Appearance	Area of dark on T1 in midbrain Area of white on T2 in midbrain, usually unilateral
Contrast	Dependent on radiologist

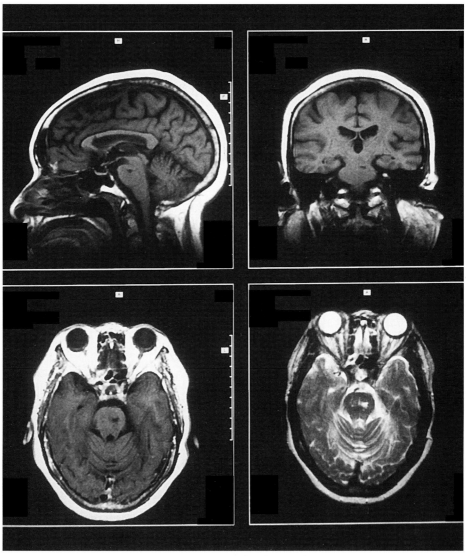

Figure 2–24 Left midbrain infarct
Upper left: T1 sagittal
Upper right: T1 coronal
Lower left: T1 axial
Lower right: T2 axial

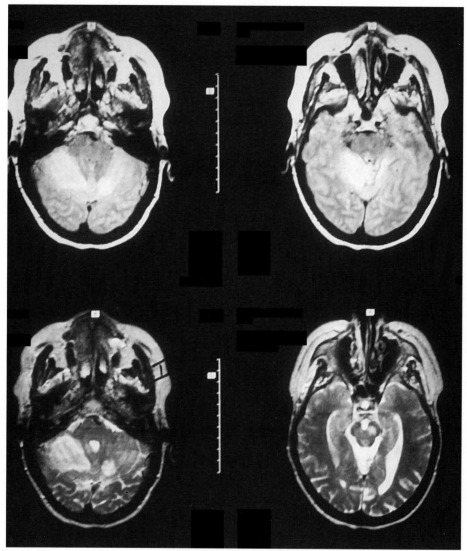

Figure 2-25 Left midbrain infarct
Right cerebellar infarct
Upper left: proton density axial
Upper right: proton density axial
Lower left: T2 axial
Lower right: T2 axial

Chart 2–16. **Head and Neck** (Fig. 2–26)

Pathology	Small vessel white matter disease
Description	Chronic ischemic changes in affected area of white matter
Symptoms	Forgetfulness Dementia Possibly asymptomatic, depending on extent of disease process
Suggested protocols	Routine brain
Appearance	Small areas of white in the white matter: T2 Not well visualized on T1
Contrast	Dependent on radiologist

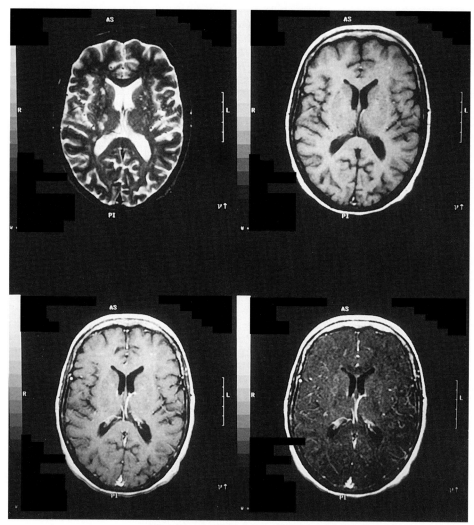

Figure 2–26 Small vessel white matter disease
Upper left: T2 axial
Upper right: T1 axial
Lower left: T1 axial (contrast)
Lower right: T1 axial (contrast)

Chart 2–17. **Head and Neck** (Figs. 2–27 and 2–28)

Pathology	Cysticercosis
Description	Parasitic disease in the brain as a result of the invasion of the larval form of the pork tapeworm
Symptoms	Seizures Headaches
Suggested protocols	Routine brain Thin slices in area of larva T1 and T2 images (multiplanar)
Appearance	Area of edema (white) surrounding larvae on T2 Area of edema (dark) surrounding larvae on T1 Possibly identify larvae in center of edema
Contrast	To show actual area of infection in brain

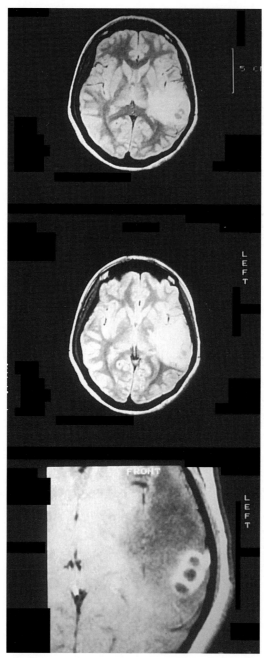

Figure 2–27 Cysticercosis
T2 axials

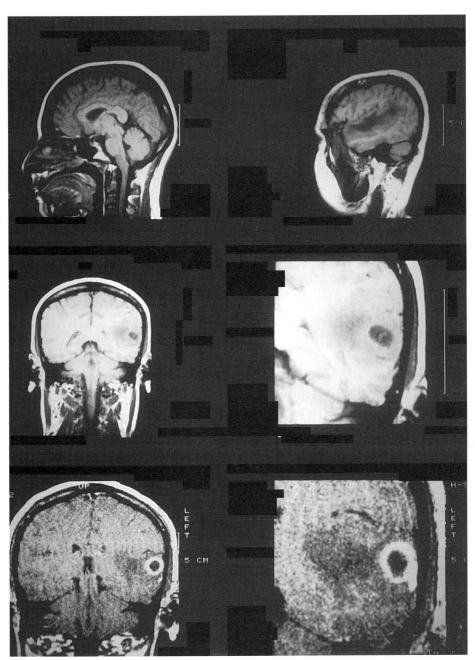

Figure 2–28 Cysticercosis
Upper: T1 sagittal
Middle left: T1 coronal
Middle right: T1 coronal (magnification)
Lower left: T1 coronal (contrast)
Lower right: T1 coronal (contrast) (magnification)

Chart 2–18. **Head and Neck** (Fig. 2–29)

Pathology	Mucormycosis
Description	Fungal infection with invasion into the orbits
Symptoms	Dependent on location Blurred vision, headaches, fever
Suggested protocols	Routine brain
Appearance	Signal void (black) from previous surgery
Contrast	To check for active infectious process

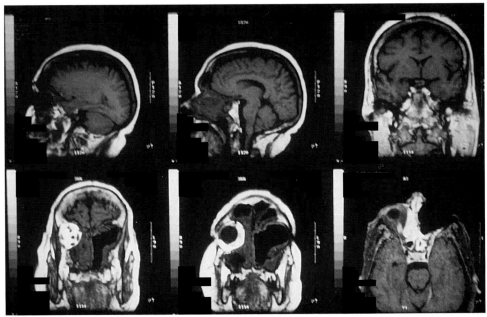

Figure 2-29 Mucormycosis
Upper left: T1 sagittal
Upper middle: T1 sagittal
Upper right: T1 coronal
Lower left: T1 coronal
Lower middle: T1 coronal
Lower right: T1 axial

Chart 2–19. **Head and Neck** (Fig. 2–30)

Pathology	Agenesis corpus callosum
Description	The corpus callosum—a white matter tract—fails to develop in the embryo, leading to complete absence of the structure in the adult
Symptoms	Asymptomatic to severe retardation
Suggested protocols	Routine brain
Appearance	Corpus callosum sitting above ventricle system is absent Absence clearly noted on sagittals
Contrast	Dependent on radiologist

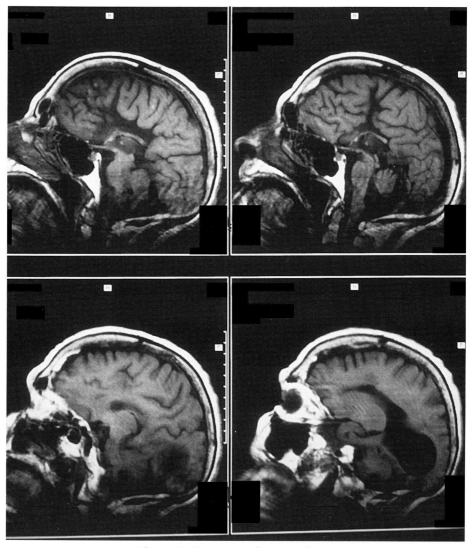

Figure 2–30 Agenesis of corpus callosum
T1 sagittals

Chart 2–20. **Head and Neck** (Figs. 2–31 to 2–34)

Pathology	Arteriovenous malformation (AVM) Aneurysm
Description	AVM: Tangle of abnormal vessels with varying diameters that have large feeding arteries and large draining veins; occurs mostly in cerebral hemisphere Aneurysm: Localized abnormal dilatation of an artery; in the head, usually are "berry" aneurysms, which occur in the bifurcations of the vessels in the circle of Willis; diameter smaller than 1.5 cm (aneurysm noted in Figs. 2–31 to 2–34 is on the middle cerebral artery)
Symptoms	AVM: Headache Patient hears pulsing in the ear Aneurysm: Headaches
Suggested protocols	Routine brain Thin slices through AVM and aneurysm MR angiography sequences through AVM and circle of Willis to obtain maximum intensity projections (arteriogram-like images)
Appearance	AVM: Cluster of black vessels on T1 Cluster of white vessels on T2 Aneurysm: Bubble of black on T1 Bubble of white on T2
Contrast	Dependent on radiologist

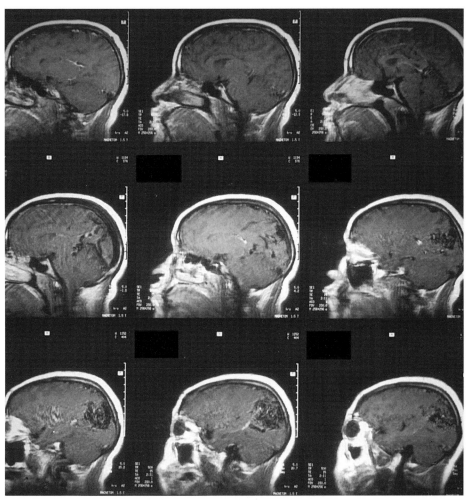

Figure 2–31 Arteriovenous malformation
Aneurysm
T1 sagittals

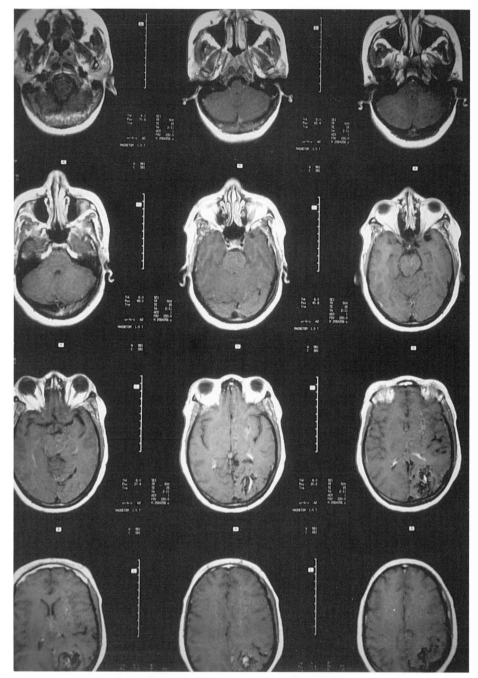

Figure 2–32 Arteriovenous malformation
Aneurysm
T1 axials

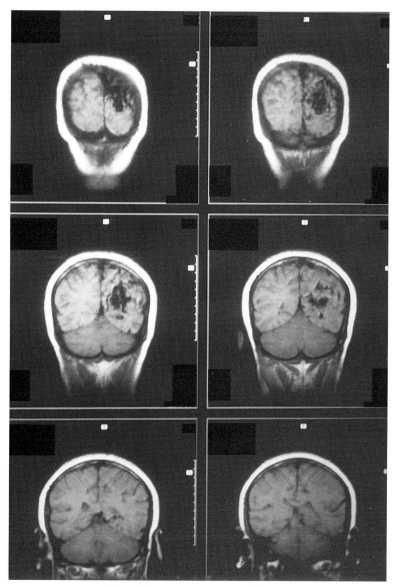

Figure 2–33 Arteriovenous malformation
Aneurysm
T1 coronals

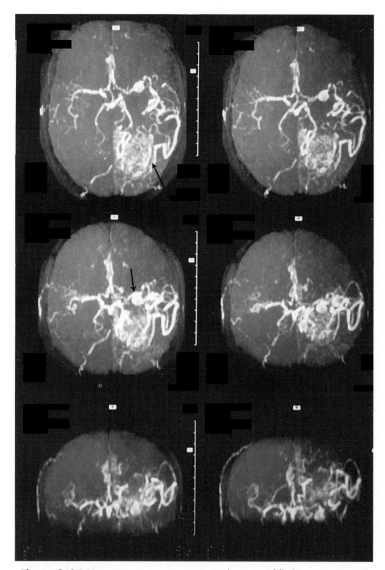

Figure 2-34 Magnetic resonance angiography, time of flight postprocessed Circle of Willis with arteriovenous malformation and middle cerebral artery aneurysm

Chart 2–21. **Head and Neck** (Fig. 2–35)

Pathology	Superior sagittal sinus (SSS) thrombus
Description	Could cause a stroke but brain's venous system has many collaterals; occlusion of a large vein produces symptoms. SSS thrombus occurs in malnourished or chronically ill people
Symptoms	Various neurologic symptoms from edema, hemorrhage, or infarction of either cerebral hemisphere
Suggested protocols	MR angiography to examine venous system Phasing out arterial flow
Appearance	Discontinuity of venous system
Contrast	Dependent on radiologist

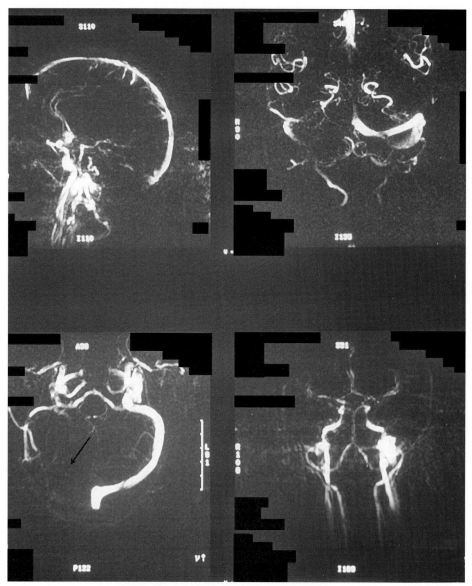

Figure 2–35 Superior sagittal sinus thrombus
Upper left: sagittal view of venous drainage
Upper right: axial view of venous drainage
Lower left: axial view of venous drainage
Lower right: coronal view of venous drainage

Chart 2–22. **Head and Neck** (Fig. 2–36)

Pathology	Nonpatent basilar artery Extra trigeminal artery on right
Description	Congenital anomaly with trigeminal artery persisting to supply posterior circulation
Symptoms	Incidental finding Headaches
Suggested protocols	Routine head Routine MRA of circle of Willis
Appearance	On MRA, basilar artery not seen, but extra vessel seen providing posterior circulation
Contrast	Dependent on radiologist

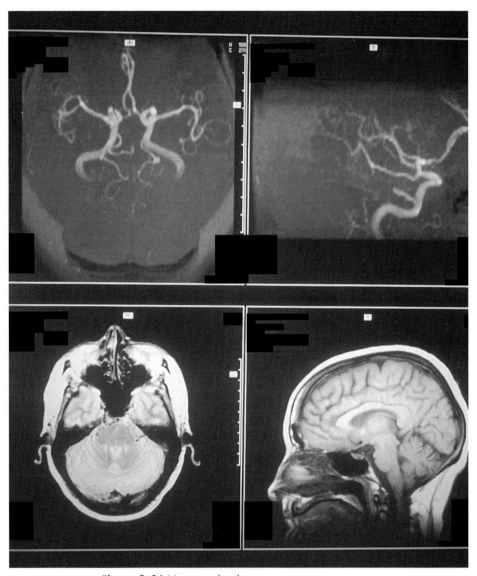

Figure 2-36 Nonpatent basilar artery
Extra trigeminal artery on right
Upper left: axial magnetic resonance angiogram (MRA)
Upper right: sagittal MRA
Lower left: T1 axial
Lower right: T1 sagittal

Chart 2–23. **Head and Neck** (Figs. 2–37 and 2–38)

Pathology	Orbit lesion
Description	Differential could be malignant melanoma or retinoblastoma. (Melanoma discussed with Fig. 2–17); retinoblastoma occurs mainly in children younger than 5 years; lesion arises from the retina and could end up extending throughout subarachnoid space
Symptoms	Visual problems
Suggested protocols	Routine head Fat saturation sequences to make normal fat around the eyeball appear dark to obtain a detailed look at the globe of the eye, nerve, and muscles. Each MRI vendor has completely different sequences to accomplish this. FOV = 200 mm; slice thickness = 3 mm, axials, coronals, and sagittals
Appearance	Lesion will appear dark in the white globe of the eye on fat saturation sequences
Contrast	Depends on lesion's visualization

FOV = field of view.

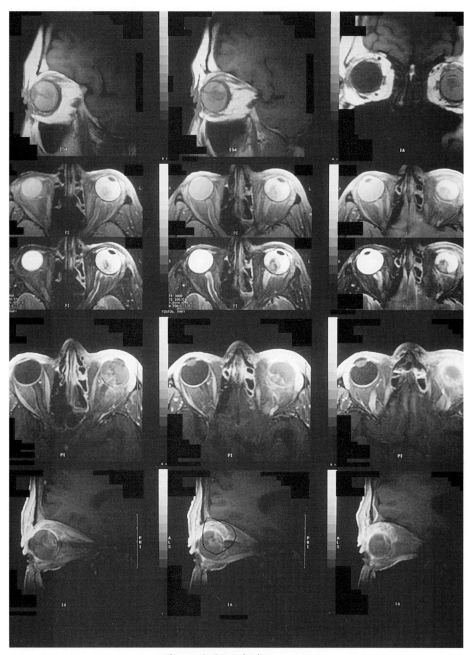

Figure 2-37 Orbit lesion
Upper left: fat saturation sagittal
Middle: fat saturation sagittal
Upper right: fat saturation coronal
Middle: fat saturation axials
Lower row: fat saturation sagittals

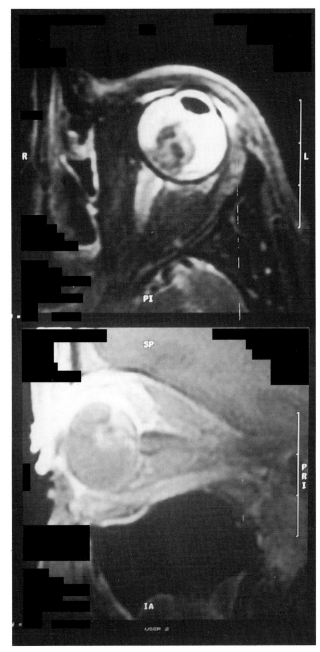

Figure 2-38 Orbit lesion
Upper: fat saturation axial
Lower: fat saturation sagittal

Chart 2–24. **Head and Neck** (Fig. 2–39)

Pathology	Parotid cysts
Description	Cysts (fluid filled) develop in the gland that sits in front of and below the ear; it secretes saliva through Stensen's duct into the mouth; cysts could cause pressure on the facial nerve
Symptoms	Fullness in area Problems with saliva production Pain around ear area Facial numbness
Suggested protocols	Routine neck
Appearance	Dark (fluid) on T1 White (fluid) on T2 Gray on proton density
Contrast	To differentiate from other lesions

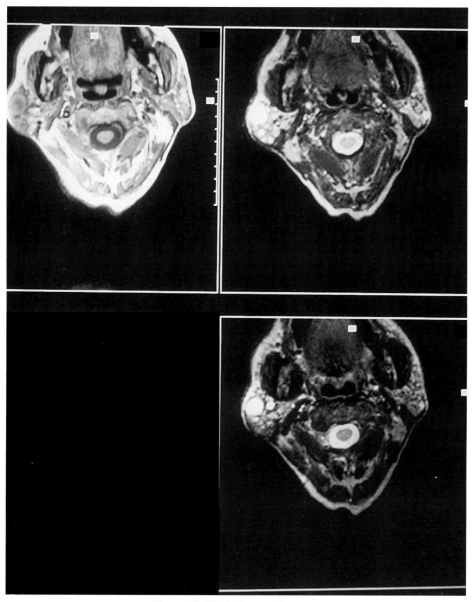

Figure 2–39 Neck, parotid cysts
Upper left: proton density axial
Upper right: T2 axial
Lower right: T2 axial

Chart 2–25. **Head and Neck** (Fig. 2–40)

Pathology	Neck abscess (prevertebral)
Description	An area of bacterial inflammation containing pus that becomes walled off
Symptoms	Redness, swelling, heat, and pain in the localized area
Suggested protocols	Routine neck
Appearance	White on T2 Irregular signal from affected tissue area
Contrast	To enhance areas of acute inflammation

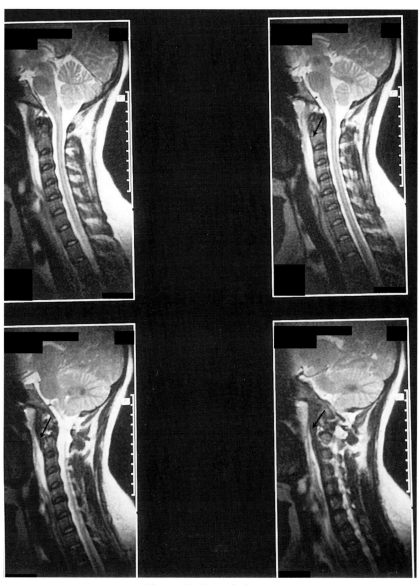

Figure 2–40 Neck abscess
T2 sagittals

Chart 2–26. **Head and Neck** (Fig. 2–41)

Pathology	Stenosis of right internal carotid artery
Description	Stenosis is narrowing of the vessel's lumen, usually from atherosclerosis; in the carotids, this does not allow adequate blood supply to the brain
Symptoms	Transient ischemic attacks Dizziness Could cause a stroke if not treated
Suggested protocols	Routine carotids using MR angiography techniques
Appearance	Narrowed vessels on MR angiographic images (postprocessed from raw data images)
Contrast	Dependent on radiologist

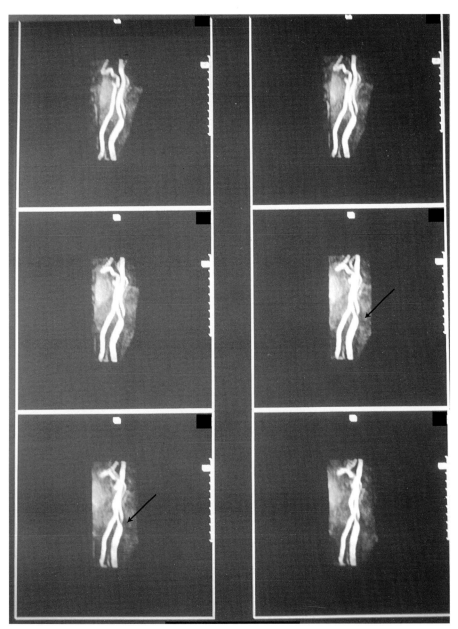

Figure 2–41 Right carotid stenosis
Magnetic resonance angiogram images showing 95%
stenosis of the right carotid

Chart 2–27. **Head and Neck** (Fig. 2–42)

Pathology	Meningioma
Description	Extra-axial benign lesion arising outside brain tissue with an attachment to dura; may infiltrate into bone and scalp and be palpable; occurs most commonly in middle-aged women
Symptoms	Motor deficits, compression of cranial nerve tracts, visual defects, all depending on location of lesion
Suggested protocols	Routine head
Appearance	Isointense on T1, T2, and proton density scans
Contrast	To actually visualize the entire lesion

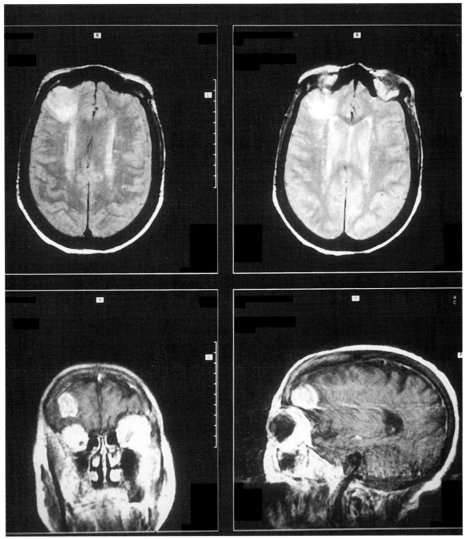

Figure 2–42 Meningioma
Upper left: T2 axial
Upper right: proton density axial
Lower left: T1 coronal (contrast)
Lower right: T1 sagittal (contrast)

CHAPTER THREE

Spine

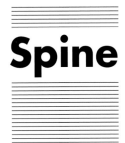

Chart 3–1. Spine (Fig. 3–1)

Pathology	Cervical Rheumatoid arthritis (RA) involvement to C1–2
Description	RA is systemic, causing erosion of articular cartilage of bone; scar tissue forms and turns to bone, thereby sometimes fusing ends of bones, causing ankylosis
Symptoms	Pain, stiffness, unable to move head very well
Suggested protocols	Routine cervical
Appearance	Irregular bone shape of C1–2 Fusion of bony end plates Irregularities: dark on T1 and T2 images
Contrast	Dependent on radiologist

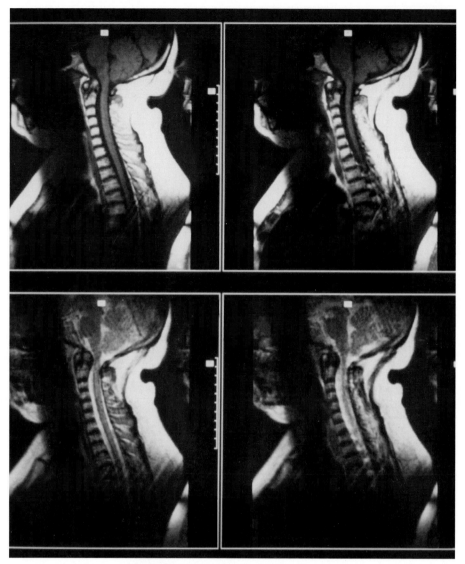

Figure 3–1 Cervical rheumatoid involvement
Upper left: T1 sagittal
Upper right: T1 sagittal
Lower left: T2 sagittal
Lower right: T2 sagittal

Chart 3-2. **Spine** (Fig. 3-2)

Pathology	Cervical stenosis
Description	Reduction of available space in the spinal column, causing compression of neural elements; could be due to growth of osteophytes and the degeneration of bones as a result of the aging process
Symptoms	Myelopathic symptoms: stenosis can cause pressure on cord and create changes in the white matter, leading to neurologic deficits; pain and stiffness
Suggested protocols	Routine cervical
Appearance	Narrowed diameter of spinal canal Narrowed disc height Dark appearance of osteophytes Gray spinal cord could have increased intensity as a result of white matter changes from chronic compression
Contrast	None

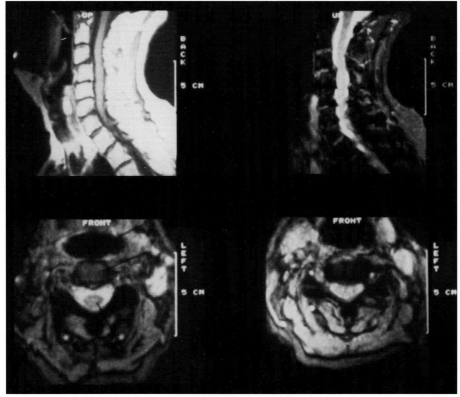

Figure 3–2 Cervical stenosis
Upper left: T1 sagittal
Upper right: T2 sagittal
Lower left: T2 axial
Lower right: T2 axial

Chart 3–3. **Spine** (Fig. 3–3)

Pathology	Cervical spurs
Description	Spicules of bone projecting into neural foramen, causing cord or nerve root compression
Symptoms	Pain in neck radiating down either arm Numbness and tingling in arms
Suggested protocols	Routine cervical
Appearance	Spicule of bone appears dark on T1 and T2 images pressing into dark or white cerebrospinal fluid surrounding spinal cord and nerve roots
Contrast	None

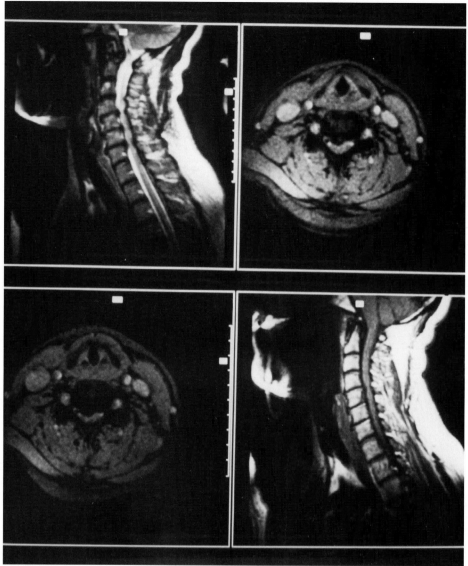

Figure 3–3 Cervical spur-disc
Upper left: T2 sagittal
Upper right: T2 axial
Lower left: T2 axial
Lower right: T1 sagittal

Chart 3–4. **Spine** (Figs. 3–4 to 3–6)

Pathology	C5–6 disc herniation
Description	Disc material (nucleus pulposus) ruptures through a tear in the annulus fibrosus
Symptoms	Pain radiating from neck down either arm, depending on location of herniation; disc pressing on nerve roots or cord could cause inflammation in the area also
Suggested protocols	Routine cervical
Appearance	Protruding disc material (nucleus pulposus) whiter, with outline of darkness representing annulus fibrosis on T1. On T2 protruding disc material is dark, pressing on white cerebrospinal fluid and gray spinal cord
Contrast	If postoperative, then contrast given to view possible scar tissue from surgery; scar tissue enhances, whereas normal disc material does not

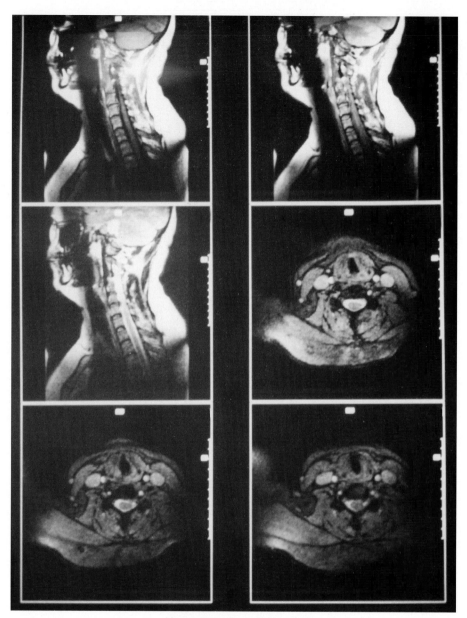

Figure 3–4 C5–6 disc herniation
Upper left: T1 sagittal
Upper right: T1 sagittal
Middle left: T2 sagittal
Middle right: T2 axial
Lower left: T2 axial
Lower right: T2 axial

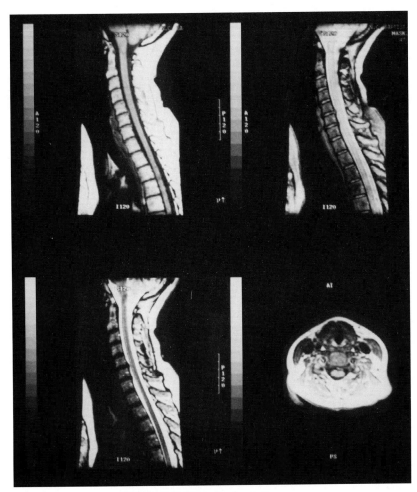

Figure 3–5 C5–6 disc herniation
Upper left: T1 sagittal
Upper right: proton density sagittal
Lower left: T2 sagittal
Lower right: T1 axial

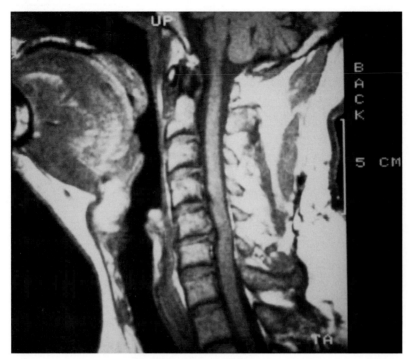

Figure 3–6 C5–6 disc herniation
T1 sagittal

Chart 3–5. **Spine** (Fig. 3–7)

Pathology	Cervical syrinx
Description	Cystic space within cord; could be caused by spinal cord lesion or Arnold-Chiari malformation (lengthening of the medulla, allowing the fourth ventricle foramina to open below the level of the foramen magnum)
Symptoms	Neurologic deficits, depending on location of syrinx; interrupt nerve tracts of pain, temperature, and gait
Suggested protocols	Routine cervical
Appearance	Syrinx appears white in the middle of the gray spinal cord on T2 images and dark in the middle of the gray spinal cord on T1 images
Contrast	To locate possible spinal cord lesion causing syrinx

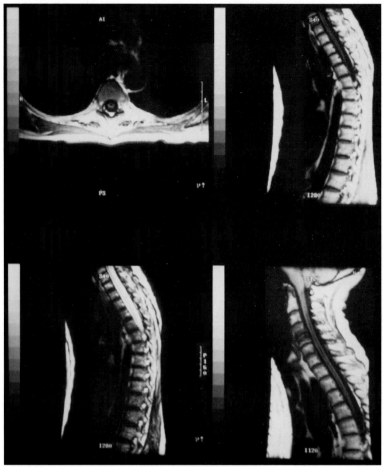

Figure 3-7 Cervical syrinx
Upper left: T1 axial
Upper right: T1 sagittal
Lower left: T2 sagittal
Lower right: T1 sagittal

Chart 3–6. **Spine** (Fig. 3–8)

Pathology	Lesion at C1–2
Description	Invasive lesion extending into bone marrow of vertebral body
Symptoms	Head and neck pain and stiffness Pain radiating down back of neck
Suggested protocols	Routine cervical Axials from the top of C-1 down to T-2
Appearance	Lesion appears dark on T1 and white on T2
Contrast	To visualize lesion and its borders

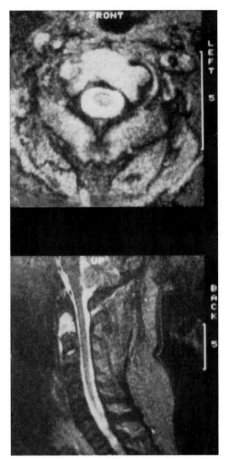

Figure 3–8 Lesion at C1–2
Upper: T2 axial
Lower: T2 sagittal

Chart 3–7. **Spine** (Fig. 3–9)

Pathology	Astrocytoma (glioma)
Description	Intramedullary malignant lesion of the central nervous system that infiltrates and grows slowly to form a firm, ill-defined mass; impossible to excise completely because of irregular borders; can have cystic components
Symptoms	Neck pain, leg and arm weakness, motor deficits
Suggested protocols	Routine cervical
Appearance	On T1 real lesion component blends in with cord; cystic components are dark On T2 all lesion components appear white
Contrast	To differentiate solid versus cystic components

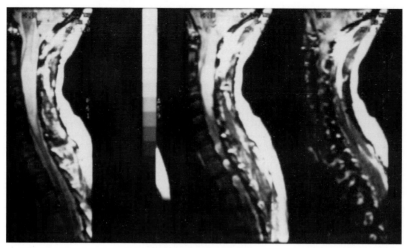

Figure 3–9 Astrocytoma
T2 sagittals

Chart 3–8. **Spine** (Fig. 3–10)

Pathology	Transection of the thoracic cord
Description	Spinal cord has been cut or severed; therefore, no communication tract for nerve fibers
Symptoms	History of severe trauma Numbness below level of transection Uncontrolled actions below level of transection
Suggested protocols	Routine thoracic Axials through level of transection to obtain complete diagnosis
Appearance	Break in normal signal or gray of spinal cord on T1 and T2
Contrast	None

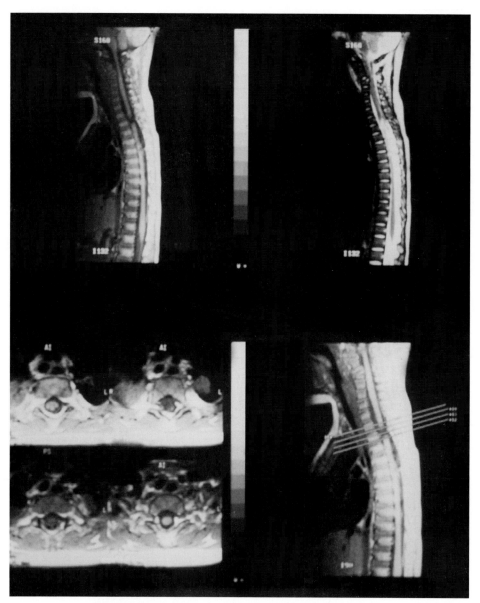

Figure 3-10 Thoracic transection of cord resulting from trauma
Upper left: T1 sagittal
Upper right: T2 sagittal
Lower left: T1 axials
Lower right: T1 sagittal

Chart 3-9. **Spine** (Figs. 3-11 and 3-12)

Pathology	Metastases to thoracic spine
Description	Cells from a primary cancer infiltrate the bone marrow of vertebral bodies and can even invade and compress the spinal cord; most common metastases to the spine are from breast and lung cancers
Symptoms	Loss of function of legs and arms, depending on level of invasion of spinal cord Numbness and pain
Suggested protocols	Routine thoracic with axials through affected levels
Appearance	Lesions appear dark in the bone marrow on T1 and whitish on T2
Contrast	To show soft tissue and bone marrow components of the metastases

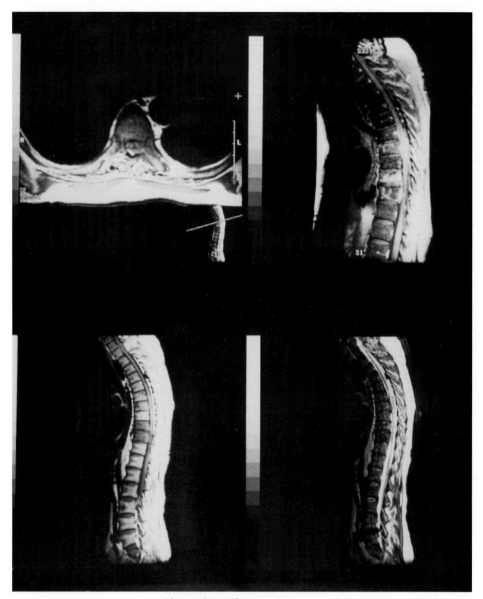

Figure 3-11 Thoracic metastases
Upper left: T1 axial
Upper right: T1 sagittal
Lower left: T1 sagittal
Lower right: T2 sagittal

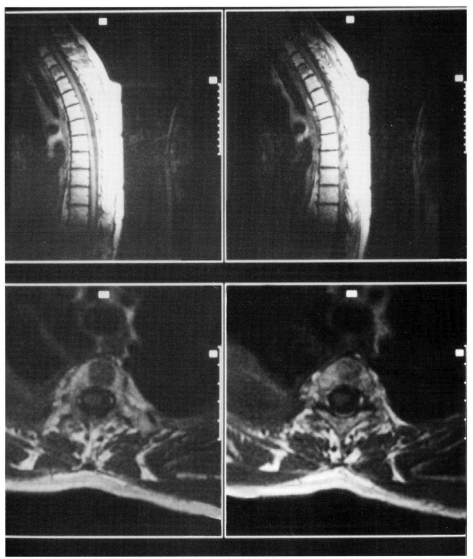

Figure 3–12 T-2 metastases
Upper left: T1 sagittal
Upper right: T1 sagittal
Lower left: T1 axial
Lower right: T1 axial

Chart 3–10. **Spine** (Fig. 3–13)

Pathology	Lesion outside cord at level of T-4, causing syrinx
Description	Probable intradural-extramedullary lesion along meninges as a result of metastases; causing syrinx (cystic cavity within spinal cord)
Symptoms	Pain Neurologic symptoms such as numbness or tingling in arms and legs from pressure on spinal canal History of cancer
Suggested protocols	Routine thoracic Axials after contrast through lesion
Appearance	Lesion not visualized until contrast given Syrinx appears dark in the gray spinal cord on T1 and white in the gray spinal cord on T2
Contrast	To examine level and borders of lesion

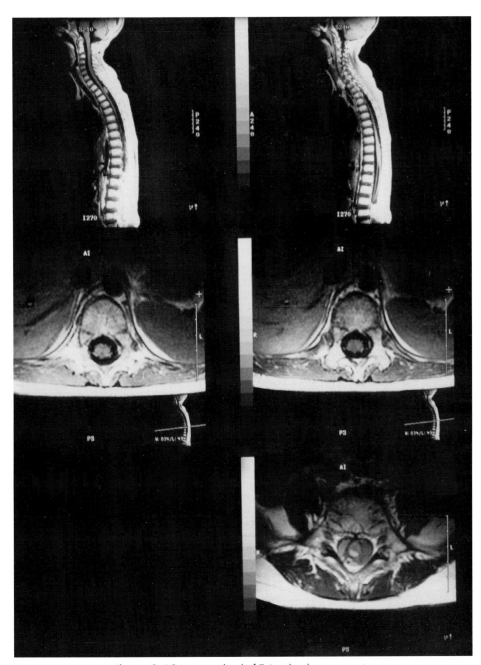

Figure 3–13 Lesion at level of T-4 with subsequent syrinx
Upper left: T1 sagittal (contrast)
Upper right: T1 sagittal
Middle left: T1 axial (contrast)
Middle right: T1 axial (contrast)
Lower right: T1 axial (contrast)

Chart 3–11. **Spine** (Fig. 3–14)

Pathology	Thoracic syrinx
Description	Fluid-filled cavity within spinal cord commonly caused by a spinal cord lesion or Arnold-Chiari malformation (lengthening of medulla, allowing fourth ventricle foramina to open below level of foramen magnum)
Symptoms	Neurologic deficits, depending on levels of thoracic cord affected; problems walking and controlling arms and legs as a result of syrinx pressing on nerve fiber tracts
Suggested protocols	Routine thoracic Axials through syrinx to check extension
Appearance	Syrinx appears dark within gray spinal cord on T1 and white within gray spinal cord on T2
Contrast	To define cause of syrinx with enhancement of possible lesion

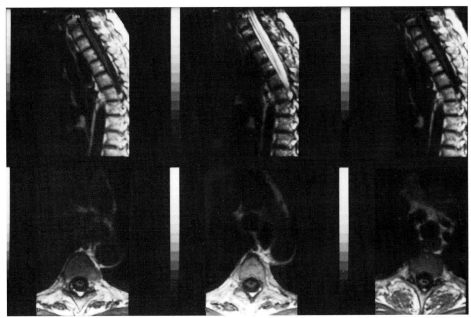

Figure 3–14 Thoracic syrinx
Upper left: T1 sagittal
Upper middle: T2 sagittal
Upper right: T1 sagittal
Lower: T1 axials

Chart 3–12. **Spine** (Figs. 3–15 and 3–16)

Pathology	Thalassemia
Description	Syndrome common in persons of Mediterranean, African, and Asian ancestry; characterized by abnormal hemoglobins; onset is in early infancy
Symptoms	Severe anemia History of sickle cell anemia Growth retardation
Suggested protocols	T1 sagittals and axials T2 sagittals and axials
Appearance	Expansion of bone marrow and thinning of cortical bone; bony deformities such as an overgrowth of bone; abnormal signal from bone marrow
Contrast	Dependent on radiologist

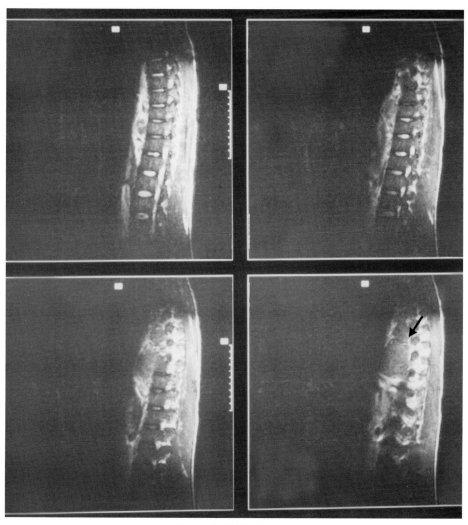

Figure 3–15 Thalassemia
T2 sagittals

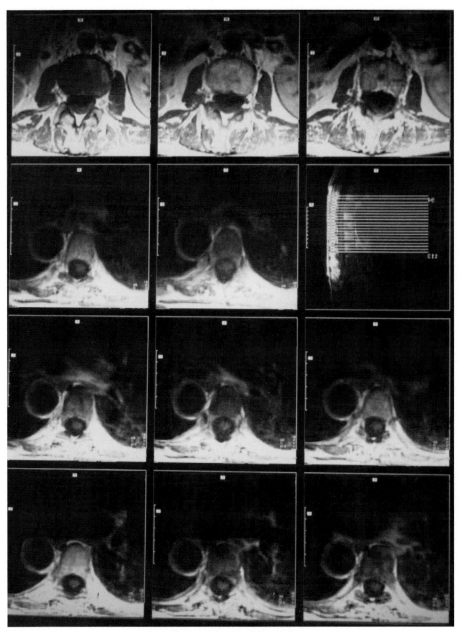

Figure 3–16 Thalassemia
T1 axials

Chart 3–13. **Spine** (Fig. 3–17)

Pathology	Lumbar collapsed disc space (after surgery)
Description	End plates of cortical bone of vertebral body are almost joined; disc space is not well differentiated; instability of level as a result of surgical intervention
Symptoms	Back pain radiating down legs
Suggested protocols	Routine lumbar
Appearance	Disc space: dark on T1 as opposed to gray of normal disc material; vertebral bodies involved could have irregular signal; darker as opposed to the normal whiter bone marrow on T1
Contrast	To visualize any acute inflammation and to enhance scar tissue, which is very vascular

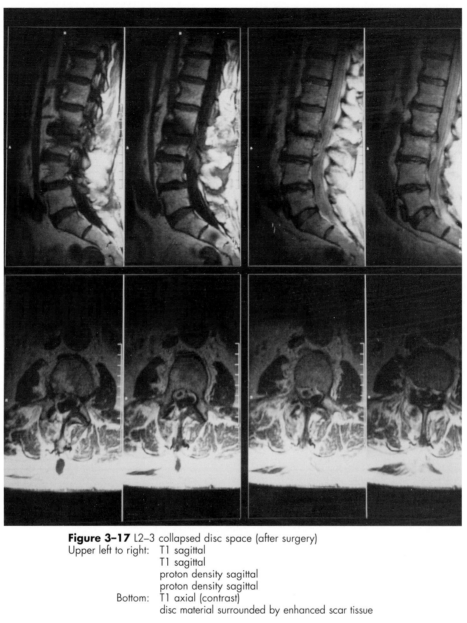

Figure 3-17 L2–3 collapsed disc space (after surgery)
Upper left to right: T1 sagittal
                       T1 sagittal
                       proton density sagittal
                       proton density sagittal
         Bottom: T1 axial (contrast)
                       disc material surrounded by enhanced scar tissue

Chart 3–14. **Spine** (Fig. 3–18)

Pathology	L-5–S-1 disc herniation
Description	Disc material (nucleus pulposus) protrudes through a tear in the outer annulus fibrosus; a bulging disc has the appearance of smooth vertebral margins; irregular margins extending beyond vertebral end plates usually indicate herniation
Symptoms	Back pain radiating down the back of either leg, depending on location of pressure from disc material
Suggested protocols	Routine lumbar
Appearance	Fat and nerve roots can be displaced (fat is white on T1 and gray on T2) Protrusion of gray disc material into white cerebrospinal fluid–filled thecal sac on T2 Protrusion of gray disc material into dark cerebrospinal fluid–filled thecal sac on T1
Contrast	If postoperative, then for scar versus disc differentiation

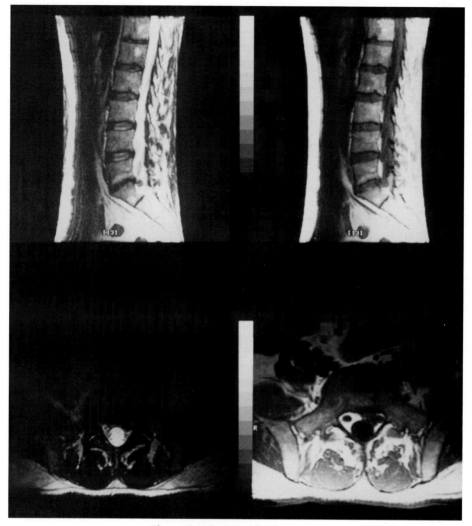

Figure 3–18 L-5–S-1 disc herniation
Upper left: T2 sagittal
Upper right: T1 sagittal
Lower left: T2 axial
Lower right: T1 axial

Chart 3–15. **Spine** (Fig. 3–19)

Pathology	Lumbar pseudomeningocele
Description	A true meningocele is usually associated with spina bifida; in a pseudomeningocele, the meningeal sac filled with cerebrospinal fluid protrudes through a vertebral defect
Symptoms	Minimal neurologic deficits Pain from surgical intervention
Suggested protocols	Routine lumbar
Appearance	Sac is white on T2 and dark on T1
Contrast	Dependent on previous surgery and radiologist

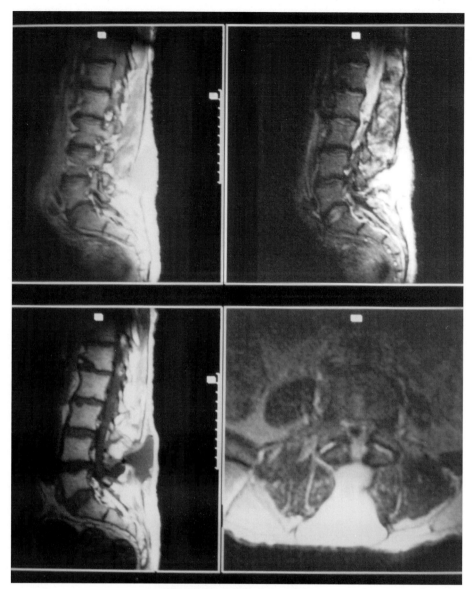

Figure 3–19 Pseudomeningocele
Upper left: proton density sagittal
Upper right: T2 sagittal
Lower left: T1 sagittal
Lower right: T2 axial

Chart 3–16. **Spine** (Fig. 3–20)

Pathology	Lumbar abnormalities Six-millimeter lesion in the subarachnoid space at L2–3 Fluid at L3–4 Spinal stenosis at L2–3
Description	Subarachnoid lesion: lesion in the space between the arachnoid and pia mater containing cerebrospinal fluid and larger blood vessels of the central nervous system Fluid (from a cerebrospinal leak or infectious process) Stenosis (narrowing of the spinal canal creating possible compression of the thecal sac)
Symptoms	Pain in back radiating down legs Stiffness Unable to walk well or sit down comfortably
Suggested protocols	Routine lumbar
Appearance	Subarachnoid lesion: gray in white cerebrospinal fluid on T2, gray in dark cerebrospinal fluid on T1; enhances well on contrast Fluid: white on T2 and dark on T1 Stenosis: spinal canal is narrowed causing compression of thecal sac usually from degenerative disc disease in the lumbar region
Contrast	To enhance lesion or infectious process

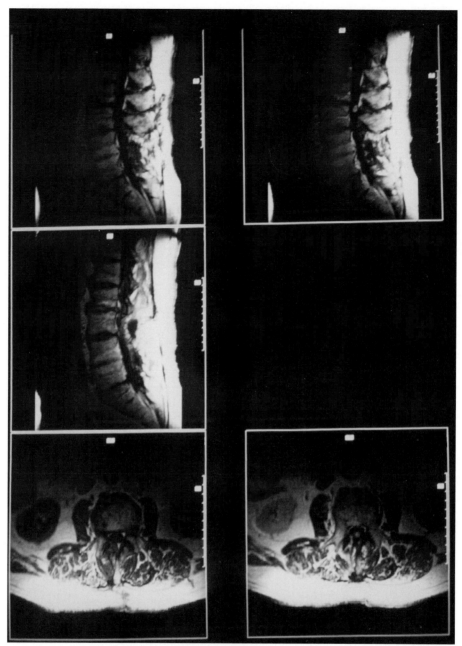

Figure 3–20 Six-mm lesion in subarachnoid space at level of L2–3
Fluid collection at L3–4
Spinal stenosis at L2–3

Upper left: T1 sagittal
Upper right: T1 sagittal
Middle: T1 sagittal (contrast)
Lower left: T1 axial
Lower right: T1 axial (contrast)

Chart 3–17. **Spine** (Fig. 3–21)

Pathology	Lumbar cerebrospinal fluid (CSF) leak
Description	Usually occurs postoperatively or after trauma. CSF leaks out into subarachnoid space from a tear in meninges
Symptoms	Headache and backache from increased pressure because of opening in the closed system of CSF around the brain and spinal cord
Suggested protocols	Routine lumbar Axials through suspect area
Appearance	CSF appears white on T2 and dark on T1
Contrast	Dependent on radiologist

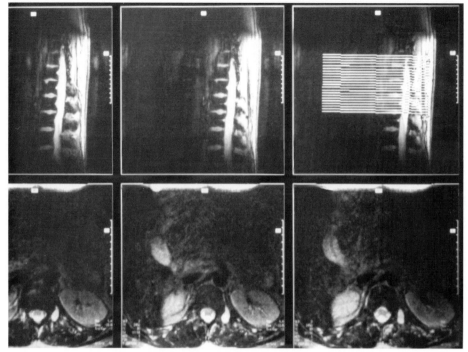

Figure 3–21 Cerebrospinal fluid leak
Upper: T2 sagittals
Lower: T2 axials

Chart 3–18. **Spine** (Fig. 3–22)

Pathology	Lipoma Tethered spinal cord Syrinx
Description	Lipoma is a fatty lesion Tethered cord results from a residual fibrous band of the cord that remains adherent to the back of the spinal canal Syrinx is a fluid-filled cavity within spinal cord
Symptoms	Lipoma: pain from pressure on nerve roots or other structures Tethered cord: incidental Syrinx: neurologic deficits, questionable spinal cord lesion or Arnold-Chiari malformation
Suggested protocols	Routine lumbar
Appearance	Lipoma appears white on T1 and gray on T2 Tethered cord appears gray and branches at level of conus and strings posteriorly Syrinx appears dark within spinal cord on T1 and white within the cord on T2
Contrast	To enhance possible lesion

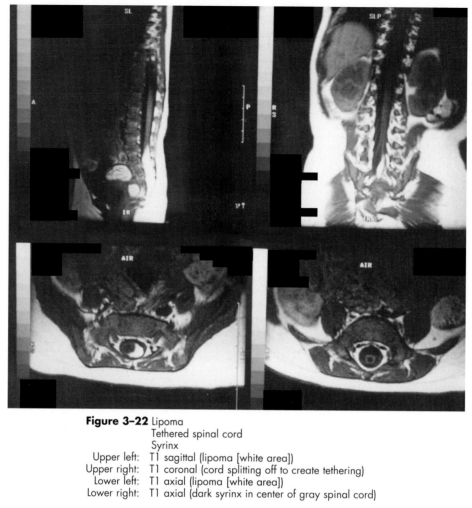

Figure 3–22 Lipoma
Tethered spinal cord
Syrinx
Upper left: T1 sagittal (lipoma [white area])
Upper right: T1 coronal (cord splitting off to create tethering)
Lower left: T1 axial (lipoma [white area])
Lower right: T1 axial (dark syrinx in center of gray spinal cord)

Chart 3–19. **Spine** (Fig. 3–23)

Pathology	Diastematomyelia
Description	Longitudinal splitting of the spinal cord at level of bony spur; common anomaly characterized by a double dural sac with associated bony spur; could be associated with a tethered cord
Symptoms	Externally on skin could see dimples and hemangiomas; leg weakness, back pain, and sensory changes
Suggested protocols	Routine thoracic or routine lumbar
Appearance	T2 appearance is of two gray, asymmetric, round, soft tissues in the white cerebrospinal fluid
Contrast	Dependent on radiologist

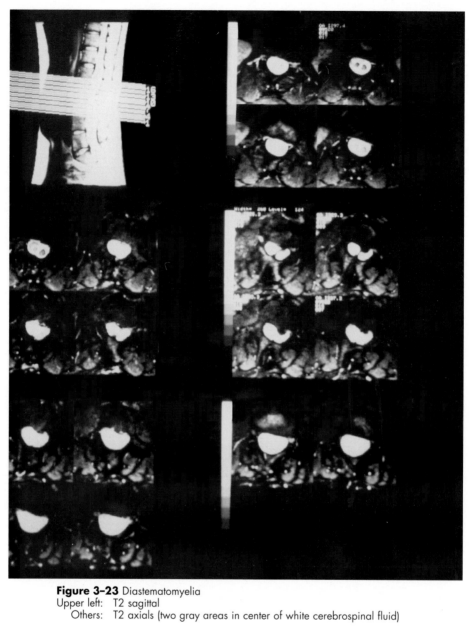

Figure 3-23 Diastematomyelia
Upper left: T2 sagittal
   Others: T2 axials (two gray areas in center of white cerebrospinal fluid)

Chart 3–20. **Spine** (Figs. 3–24 and 3–25)

Pathology	Metastases to lumbar spine
Description	Cells from a primary cancer infiltrate bone marrow of vertebral bodies with possible invasion to compress nerve roots and thecal sac, depending on level of involvement
Symptoms	Depending on level of involvement, there could be bowel and bladder changes, loss of function of legs and arms, numbness, and pain
Suggested protocols	Routine lumbar
Appearance	Metastases appear dark in the bone marrow on T1, and soft tissue parts appear gray Metastases appear whitish in the bone marrow on T2, and soft tissue parts appear gray
Contrast	To enhance metastases, including the soft tissue components

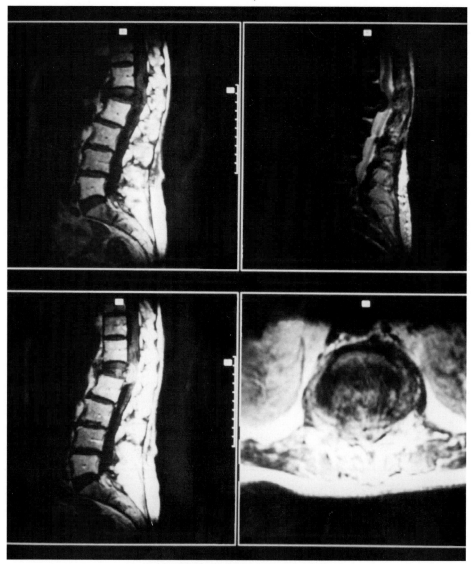

Figure 3–24 L-1 metastases to spinal cord
Upper left: T1 sagittal
Upper right: T2 sagittal
Lower left: T1 sagittal (contrast)
Lower right: T1 axial (contrast)

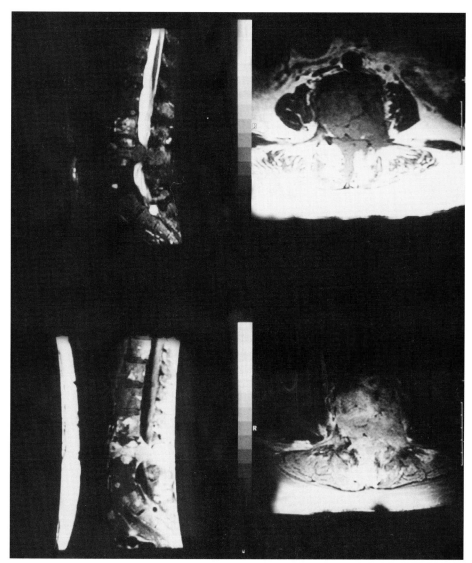

Figure 3–25 Lumbar metastases
Upper left: T2 sagittal
Upper right: T1 axial
Lower left: T1 sagittal (contrast)
Lower right: T1 axial (contrast)

CHAPTER FOUR

Body

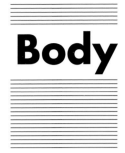

Chart 4–1. **Body** (Figs. 4–1 and 4–2)

Pathology	Coarctation of the aorta
Description	Localized narrowing of the aorta directly distal to the closed ductus arteriosus; occurs in males more than in females
Symptoms	Pain in leg muscles during exercise from inadequate blood supply and hypertension Asymptomatic if enough collateral circulation
Suggested protocols	T1 parasagittal T2 parasagittal FOV = 320 mm Slice thickness = 6–8 mm Matrix = 256 × 256
Appearance	Aortic blood flow appears white on T2 with slowed blood flow in the narrowing appearing grayish Aortic blood flow appears black on T1 with slowed blood flow in the narrowing appearing grayish
Contrast	None

FOV = field of view.

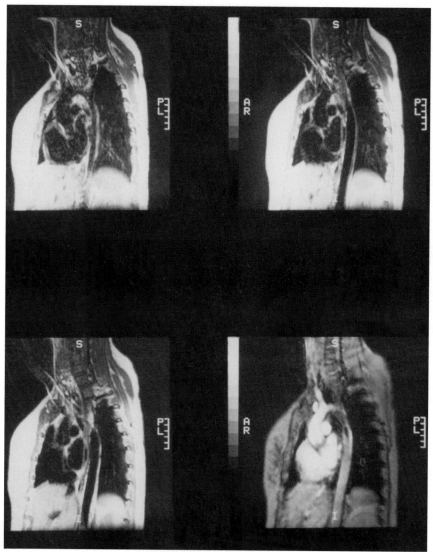

Figure 4–1 Coarctation
Upper left: T1 parasagittal
Upper right: T1 parasagittal
Lower left: T1 parasagittal
Lower right: T2 parasagittal

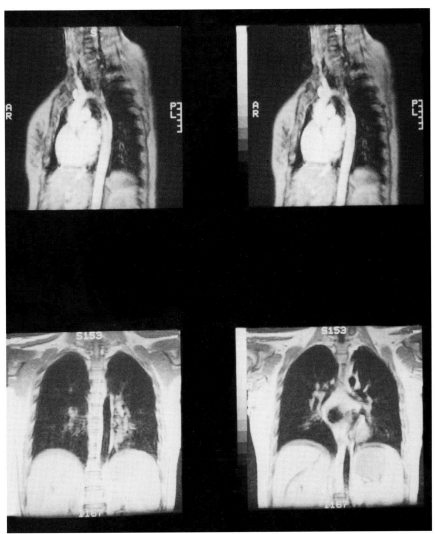

Figure 4–2 Coarctation
Upper left: T2 parasagittal
Upper right: T2 parasagittal
Lower left: T1 coronal
Lower right: T1 coronal

Chart 4–2. **Body** (Fig. 4–3)

Pathology	Thrombus in right atrium
Description	Blood clots can form in the atrial chambers when turbulence and stasis of blood occur; usually with patients who have mitral valve stenosis or atrial fibrillation; fragments can detach and form emboli in the blood stream, which can go to the lungs or to the brain
Symptoms	Murmur from stenosis of mitral valve Chest pain Increases pulmonary venous pressure Pulmonary edema
Suggested protocols	T1 sagittals and axials T2 sagittal FOV = 320 mm Slice thickness = 5–6 mm Matrix = 256 × 256
Appearance	On T1, the chambers of the heart are black from blood flow; the thrombus appears gray in the black chamber On T2, the chambers of the heart are white from blood flow; the thrombus appears gray in the white chamber
Contrast	Dependent on radiologist

FOV = field of view.

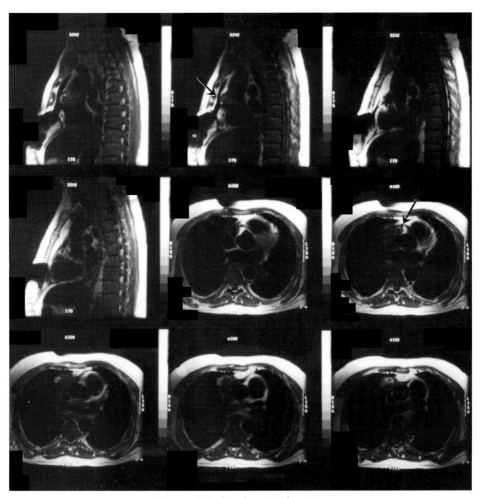

Figure 4–3 Thrombus in right atrium
Upper: T1 sagittals
Middle left: T1 sagittal
Middle center: T1 axial
Middle right: T1 axial
Lower: T1 axial

Chart 4–3. **Body** (Fig. 4–4)

Pathology	Ascending aortic aneurysm
Description	With atherosclerotic disease causing slow flow in aorta, walls weaken and dilate, causing an aneurysm
Symptoms	Chest pain, circulation problems, and increased blood pressure
Suggested protocols	Routine heart
Appearance	T1 blood flow is dark and area of slow flow appears gray; dilation of diameter of aorta
Contrast	Dependent on radiologist

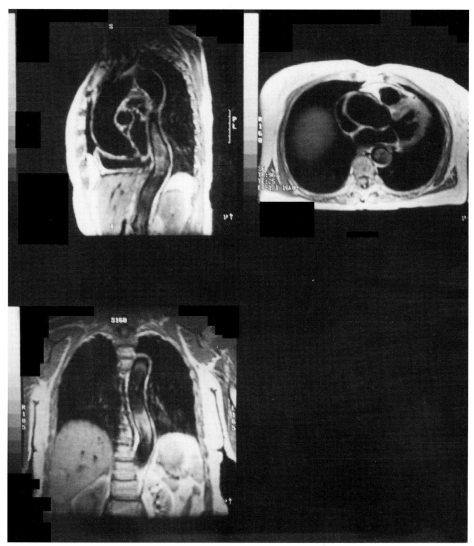

Figure 4–4 Aortic aneurysm
Upper left: T1 sagittal
Upper right: T1 axial
Lower left: T1 coronal

Chart 4-4. **Body** (Figs. 4-5 to 4-7)

Pathology	Renal cell carcinoma Fatty changes in pancreatic head
Description	Renal cell: malignant lesion that is usually solid ranging in size from small to very large Sometimes the lesion can contain small cysts Invasion into the renal vein is common with possible invasion into the inferior vena cava; metastasis to the lung, bone, liver, brain, and other organs
Symptoms	Renal: hematuria, flank pain, fever, and hypertension Pancreatic head changes: possible bile duct obstruction and duodenal displacement
Suggested protocols	T1 axials and coronals T2 axials and coronals FOV = 400 mm Slice thickness = 4–5 mm Matrix = 256 × 256
Appearance	Renal: lesion appears whiter than the gray kidney on T1 and T2 images; asymmetric kidney size Pancreatic changes: fat appears white on T1 and grayish on T2 images; pancreas should be homogeneous in appearance on all images
Contrast	To check invasiveness of lesion into other organs in abdomen

FOV = field of view.

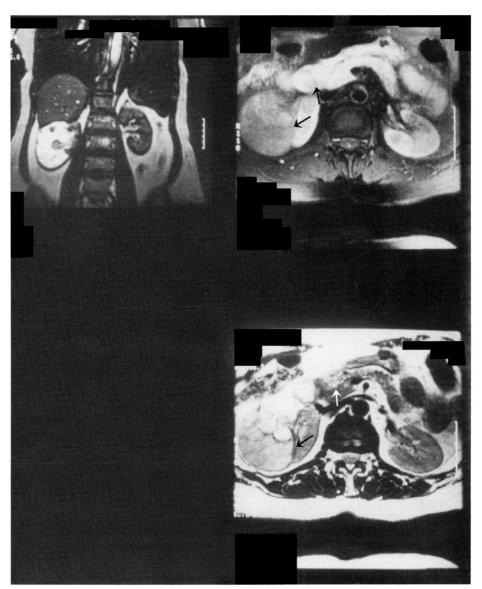

Figure 4–5 Renal cell carcinoma
Fatty changes in pancreatic head
Upper left: T2 coronal
Upper right: T2 axial
Lower: T1 axial

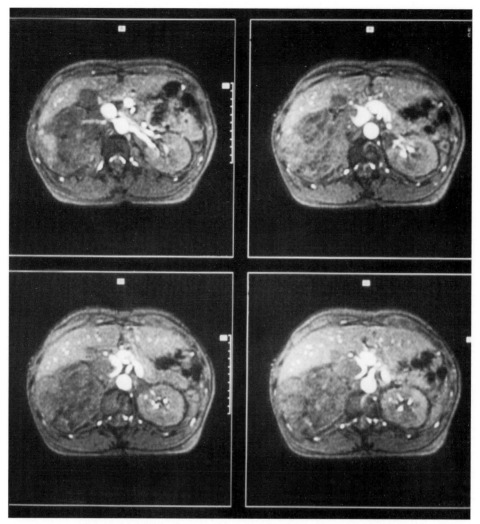

Figure 4–6 Renal cell carcinoma with invasion into inferior vena cava
T2 axials

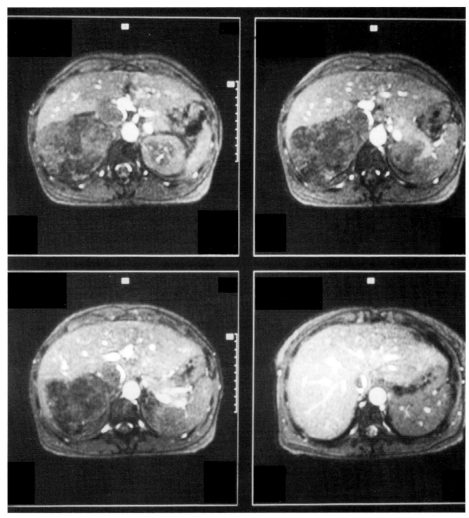

Figure 4–7 Renal cell carcinoma with invasion into inferior vena cava
T2 axials

Chart 4–5. **Body** (Fig. 4–8)

Pathology	Adrenal lesion
Description	Adrenal gland is a common site for metastases from lung cancers; if lesion is an adrenal carcinoma (a primary cancer), it is highly malignant with metastases via lymph system and blood stream
Symptoms	Hormone imbalance with menstrual irregularities in women Fatigue History of a primary cancer
Suggested protocols	T1 axials and coronals T2 axials and coronals FOV = 400 mm Slice thickness = 4–5 mm Matrix = 256 × 256
Appearance	Irregular signal (white or dark) from the small, grayish, triangular-shaped adrenal gland; abnormal size of adrenal gland
Contrast	To check for metastatic disease and lesion infiltration

FOV = field of view.

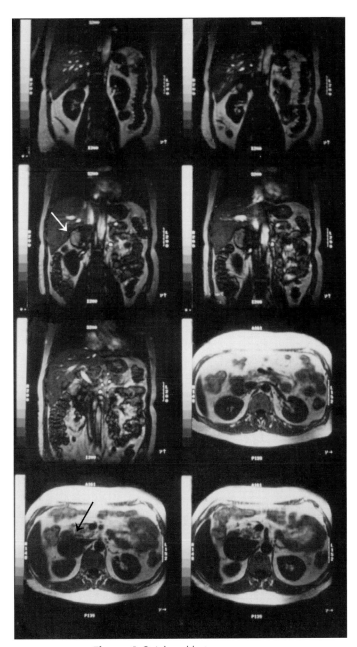

Figure 4–8 Adrenal lesion
Line 1:   T2 coronals
Line 2:   T2 coronals
Line 3:   left, T2 coronal; right, T1 axial
Line 4:   T1 axials

Chart 4–6. **Body** (Fig. 4–9)

Pathology	Psoas muscle hematoma
Description	Blood in fibers of psoas muscle
Symptoms	Flank pain History of trauma to lower back
Suggested protocols	T1 axials and coronals T2 axials and coronals
Appearance	On T1, blood appears white in the gray muscle On T2, blood appears white in the gray muscle
Contrast	To differentiate from other lesions Dependent on radiologist

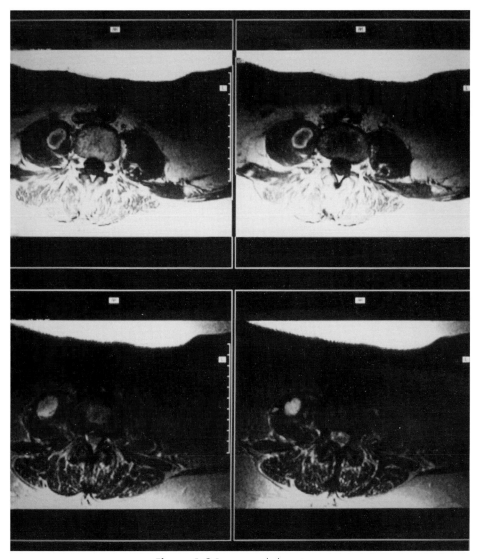

Figure 4–9 Psoas muscle hematoma
Upper left: T1 axial
Upper right: T1 axial
Lower left: T2 axial
Lower right: T2 axial

Chart 4–7. **Body** (Figs. 4–10 to 4–12)

Pathology	Breast: silicone leak
Description	Implants are placed either subglandularly or subpectorally; the body forms a capsule of scar tissue around the implant as a result of the immune response to a foreign body; most implants have an inner and outer lumen; intracapsular tears leak silicone into breast tissue in capsule (linguine sign, or string appearance); extracapsular tears leak silicone outside fibrous capsule into breast parenchyma
Symptoms	Hard, painful breast that could become misshapen
Suggested protocols	Breast coil that transmits and receives radiofrequency field Axial and sagittal T2 Slice thickness = 5–6 mm FOV = 350 mm axial and 200 mm sagittal Silicone-specific scan sequences because silicone has long T1 and T2 relaxation times Fat suppression techniques can be used for lesion visualization
Appearance	Free portion of capsule seen suspended in implant-linguine sign or free-floating loose threads
Contrast	None

FOV = field of view.

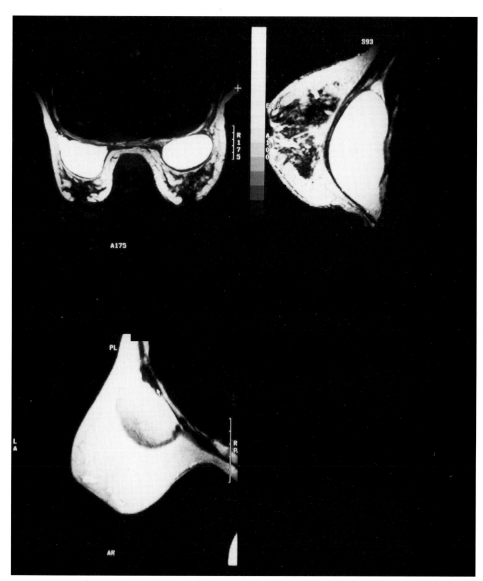

Figure 4–10 Breasts: silicone rupture
Upper left: T2 axial
Upper right: T2 sagittal
Lower: T1 off axis sagittal

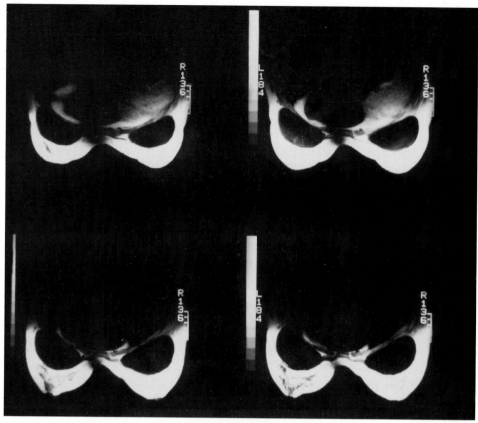

Figure 4–11 Breasts: silicone rupture
T2 axials

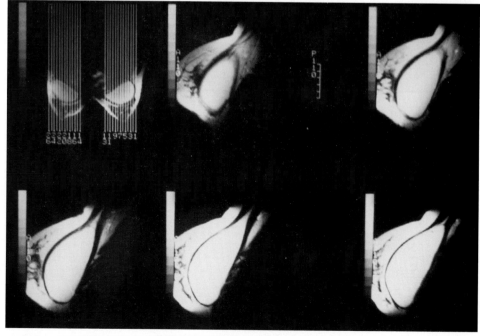

Figure 4–12 Breasts: silicone rupture
T2 sagittals

Chart 4–8. **Body** (Fig. 4–13)

Pathology	Male pelvis Blocked seminal vesicles
Description	Seminal vesicles are accessory glands near the base of the bladder that join the vas deferens to form the ejaculatory duct; they provide fructose, nutrients, and prostaglandin in their secretions for the semen
Symptoms	Problems with urination and ejaculation
Suggested protocols	Endorectal coil FOV = 130 mm Slice thickness = 3 mm Matrix = 256 × 256 T2 axials, coronals, and sagittals
Appearance	White enlarged vesicles on T2 Dark enlarged vesicles on T1
Contrast	To enhance possible lesion causing blockage

FOV = field of view.

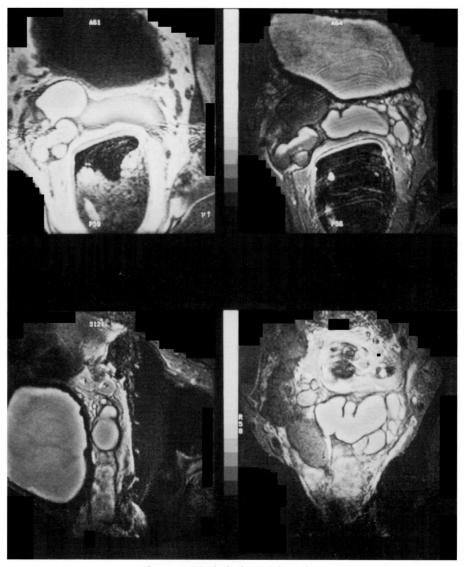

Figure 4–13 Blocked seminal vesicles
Upper left: T1 axial
Upper right: T2 axial
Lower left: T2 sagittal
Lower right: T2 coronal

Chart 4–9. **Body** (Fig. 4–14)

Pathology	Rectal lesion
Description	Probable cancer of the rectum; rectal lesions are malignant ulcers with raised everted edges
Symptoms	Asymptomatic in early stages Blood in stools Change in bowel habits
Suggested protocols	T1 axials and sagittals T2 axials and sagittals Endorectal coil can be used for better detail if in use at the facility
Appearance	Enlarged rectum displacing bladder, rectum, and prostate Lesion may appear darker than normal rectal tissue on T1 and whiter on T2
Contrast	Dependent on radiologist

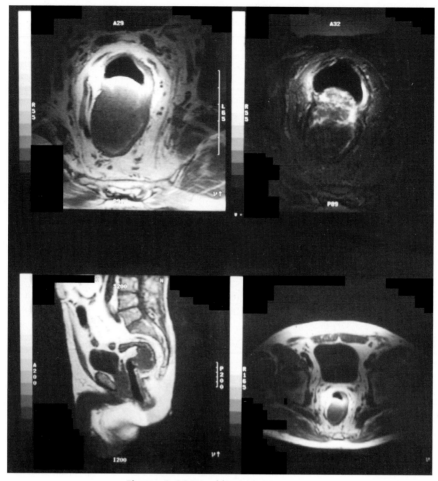

Figure 4–14 Rectal lesion
Upper left: T1 axial (endorectal coil)
Upper right: T2 axial (endorectal coil)
Lower left: T1 sagittal
Lower right: T1 axial

Chart 4–10. **Body** (Fig. 4–15)

Pathology	Uterine lesion
Description	Uterine lesion causing uterine enlargement, possible carcinoma
Symptoms	Lesions in the uterus usually reach a large size before any clinical symptoms appear Irregular bleeding
Suggested protocols	T1 axials and sagittals T2 axials and sagittals FOV = 400 mm Slice thickness = 5–6 mm Matrix = 256 × 256 Coronals if deemed necessary
Appearance	Enlarged gray uterus with possible displacement of bladder and rectum
Contrast	To check extension of lesion

FOV = field of view.

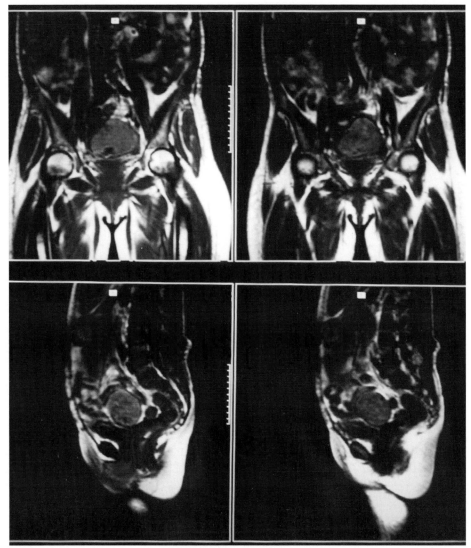

Figure 4-15 Uterine lesion
Upper left: T1 coronal
Upper right: T1 coronal
Lower left: T1 sagittal
Lower right: T1 sagittal

CHAPTER FIVE

Musculoskeletal

Chart 5–1. **Musculoskeletal** (Figs. 5–1 and 5–2)

Pathology	Temporomandibular joint (TMJ) Anterior dislocation of meniscus
Description	Meniscus (articular disc) does not return to its normal position above the mandibular condyle during opening of mouth; attempts can lead to erosion over a long period of time
Symptoms	Local pain Joint noises (clicking, popping) Earache, headache Limited jaw motion
Suggested protocols	Routine TMJ with equipment (ratchet device) to permit closed mouth imaging and opening motion of the mouth imaging
Appearance	Meniscus is black on T1 and T2 images Bow tie–shaped meniscus should sit over the mandibular condyle for normal open mouth position
Contrast	None

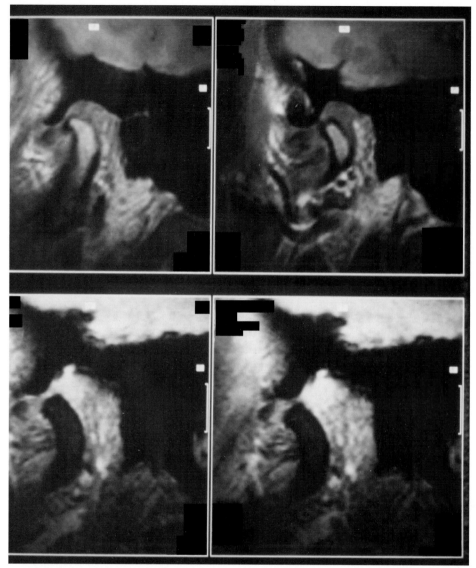

Figure 5-1 Right anterior dislocation of meniscus without reduction of temporomandibular joint
Upper left:　T1 sagittal (closed)
Upper right:　T1 sagittal (closed)
Lower left:　T2 sagittal (open without reduction)
Lower right:　T2 sagittal (open without reduction)

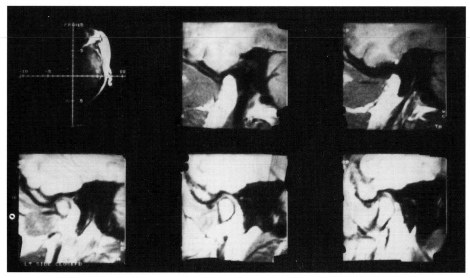

Figure 5–2 Left anterior dislocation of meniscus of temporomandibular joint
T1 sagittals (closed)

Chart 5–2. **Musculoskeletal** (Fig. 5–3)

Pathology	Rotator cuff tear
Description	Tears could occur as a result of chronic impingement of the fibers; a full tear allows communication between the glenohumeral joint and the subacromial bursa; tears commonly involve the supraspinatus tendon
Symptoms	Pain and inflammation Unable to raise arm above head
Suggested protocols	Routine shoulder
Appearance	Interruption of the tendon's black band of fibers; appears white around the tendon on T2; tendon fibers could be retracted and be free floating
Contrast	None

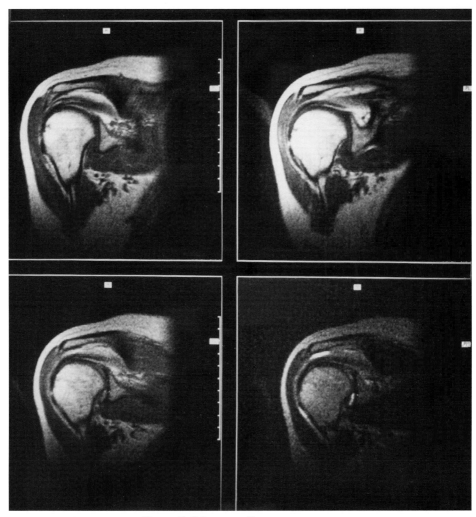

Figure 5–3 Rotator cuff tear
Upper left: T1 paracoronal
Upper right: T1 paracoronal
Lower left: proton density paracoronal
Lower right: T2 paracoronal

Chart 5–3. **Musculoskeletal** (Figs. 5–4 and 5–5)

Pathology	Metastasis to shoulder Destructive lesion of the humeral head
Description	Primary cancer lesions are rare in the shoulder; both of these lesions are aggressive as determined by the margins; metastatic deposits from primary cancer with involvement of cortical bone and bone marrow with erosion
Symptoms	Pain and swelling History of primary cancer
Suggested protocols	Routine shoulder
Appearance	Lesion appears dark on T1 and white on T2
Contrast	To delineate metastatic lesion

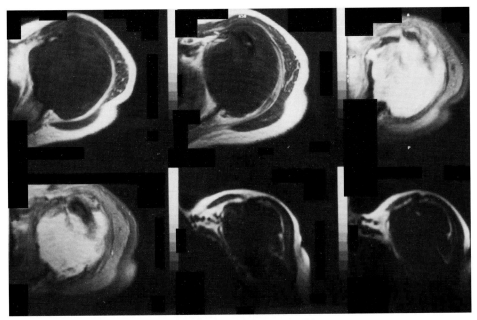

Figure 5–4 Metastases to shoulder
Upper left: T1 axial
Upper middle: T1 axial
Upper right: T2 axial
Lower left: T2 axial
Lower middle: T1 paracoronal
Lower right: T1 paracoronal

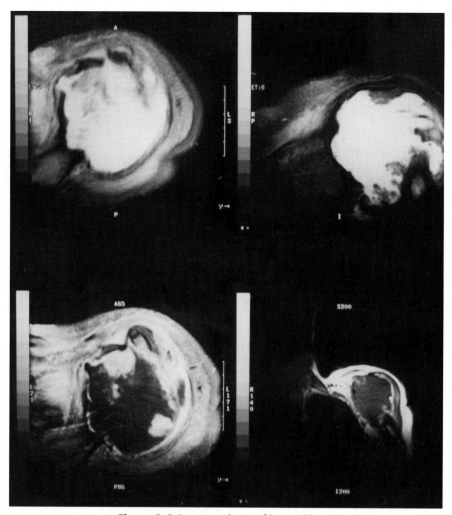

Figure 5–5 Destructive lesion of humeral head
Upper left: T2 axial
Upper right: T2 axial
Lower left: T2 axial
Lower right: T1 coronal

Chart 5–4. **Musculoskeletal** (Figs. 5–6 and 5–7)

Pathology	Hematoma around humerus
Description	Accumulation of blood and fluid in soft tissue from trauma to area
Symptoms	Pain and swelling as a result of trauma Palpable knot
Suggested protocols	T1 coronals, axials, and sagittals T2 coronals, axials, and sagittals FOV = 300 mm Slice thickness = 5 mm
Appearance	T1 fluid accumulation will appear dark T2 fluid accumulation will appear white
Contrast	To differentiate from other lesions

FOV = field of view.

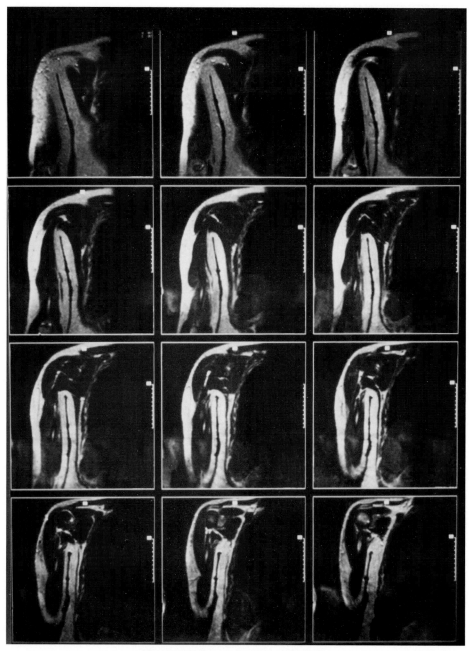

Figure 5–6 Hematoma around humerus
T2 coronals

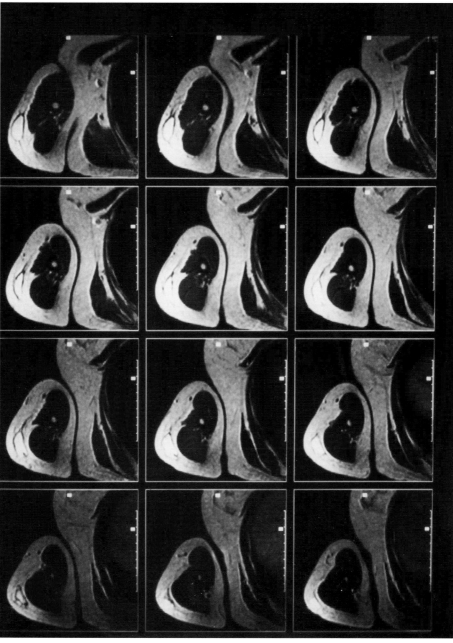

Figure 5-7 Hematoma around humerus
T2 axials

Chart 5–5. **Musculoskeletal** (Fig. 5–8)

Pathology	Osteochondritis dissecans of the elbow
Description	Partial or complete separation of articular cartilage and subchondral bone from the "mother" bone; a piece of bone becomes necrotic, occurring from repetitive trauma that damages layers of superficial bone; covering of cartilage remains intact but underneath bone is necrotic; MR is done to check for fragmentation of necrotic bone and for intact cartilage covering
Symptoms	Intermittent pain and swelling
Suggested protocols	T1 axials and coronals T2 axials and coronals Slice thickness = 3–4 mm FOV = 190 mm Matrix = 256 × 256
Appearance	Necrotic bone appears dark in whiter bone marrow on T1; on T2, pieces of necrotic bone can appear dark inside the bone marrow
Contrast	To check for possible active infection

FOV = field of view.

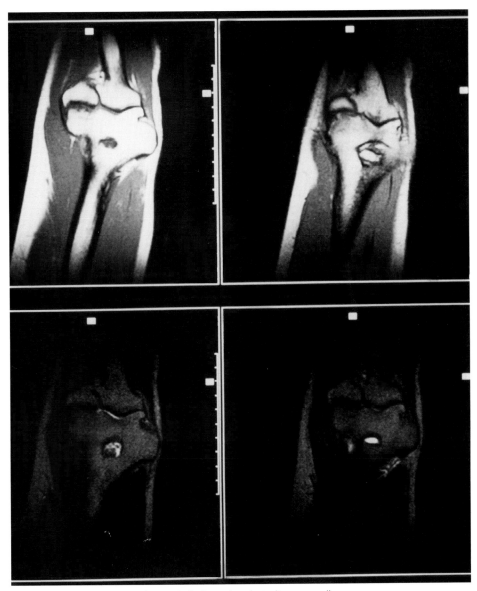

Figure 5-8 Osteochondritis dissecans, elbow
Upper left: T1 coronal
Upper right: T1 coronal
Lower left: T2 coronal
Lower right: T2 coronal

Chart 5–6. **Musculoskeletal** (Fig. 5–9)

Pathology	Distal radial lesions
Description	Differentials of the lesion include a giant cell tumor located at epiphysis in an adult; soft tissue involvement could occur; enchondroma—benign lesions in metacarpals and phalanges—and fluid-filled bone cyst are other possibilities
Symptoms	Pain and swelling Pathologic fracture
Suggested protocols	T1 axials, coronals, and sagittals T2 axials, coronals, and sagittals FOV = 140 mm Slice thickness = 3–4 mm Matrix = 192 × 256
Appearance	Dark area where lesion has invaded bone marrow on T1 and grayish on T2
Contrast	To differentiate between cyst and invasive lesion

FOV = field of view.

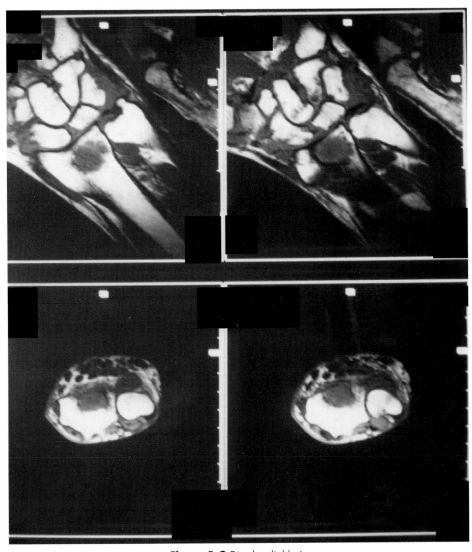

Figure 5-9 Distal radial lesion
Upper: T1 coronal
Lower: T1 axial

Chart 5–7. **Musculoskeletal** (Fig. 5–10)

Pathology	Left hip fracture
Description	Femoral neck fracture that is nondisplaced and difficult to see on plain film radiography
Symptoms	Hip pain and swelling History of trauma Unable to bear weight on hip joint
Suggested protocols	Routine hips
Appearance	Fracture line appears dark in white bone marrow on T1 and darker in grayish bone marrow on T2 images
Contrast	None unless pathologic fracture is suspected

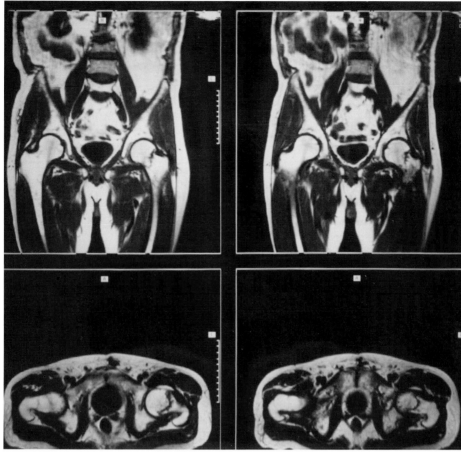

Figure 5–10 Left hip fracture
Upper left: T1 coronal
Upper right: T1 coronal
Lower left: T1 axial
Lower right: T1 axial

Chart 5–8. **Musculoskeletal** (Fig. 5–11)

Pathology	Thigh lesion
Description	Soft tissue neoplasm: benign versus malignant Biopsy used to characterize
Symptoms	Painful with swelling as lesion grows Palpable lesion
Suggested protocols	T1 axials, coronals, and sagittals T2 axials, coronals, and sagittals FOV = 300 mm Slice thickeness = 5 mm Matrix = 192 × 256
Appearance	Appearance is very similar to that of normal soft tissue, somewhat darker on T1 and whiter on T2
Contrast	To identify involvement of muscles and nerve fibers of benign or malignant lesion

FOV = field of view.

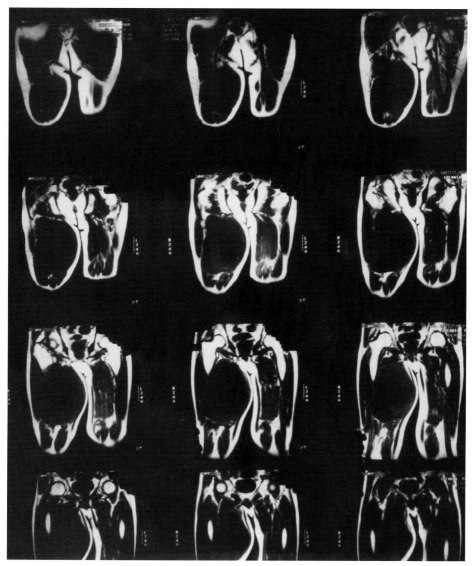

Figure 5–11 Thigh lesion
T1 coronals

Chart 5–9. **Musculoskeletal** (Figs. 5–12 and 5–13)

Pathology	Abnormal subcutaneous fat in hips, thighs, and legs
Description	Differential could be nonenzymatic fat necrosis, which occurs in subcutaneous tissue; patients could have a history of trauma; evokes inflammatory response with fibrotic tissue forming
Symptoms	Trauma with pain and swelling Palpable nodules in area
Suggested protocols	Routine hips
Appearance	On T1, fat appears white On T2, fat appears gray
Contrast	To differentiate from other lesions

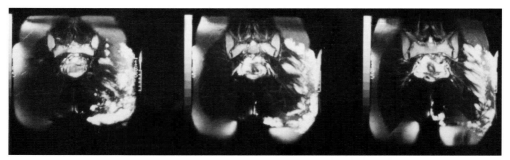

Figure 5–12 Abnormal subcutaneous fat in soft tissue
T1 coronals

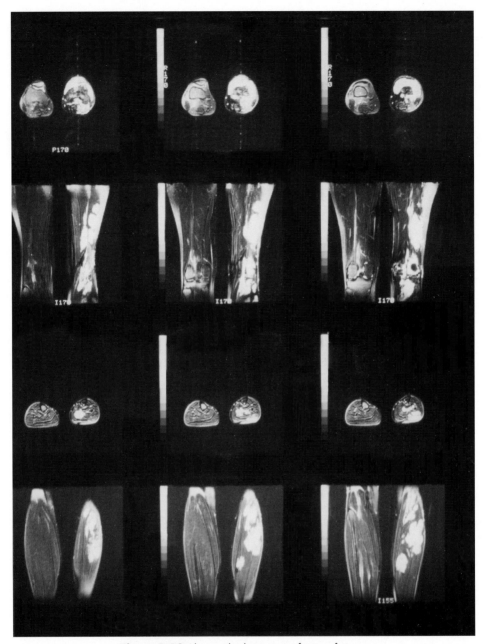

Figure 5–13 Abnormal subcutaneous fat in soft tissue
Upper row: T1 axials
Upper middle row: T1 coronals
Lower middle row: T1 axials
Lower row: T1 coronals

Chart 5–10. **Musculoskeletal** (Figs. 5–14 and 5–15)

Pathology	Knee Medial meniscus tear, posterior horn
Description	A C-shaped irregularity in the medial meniscus; its posterior horn is larger than the medial or lateral aspects; the menisci are fibrocartilaginous in nature and provide a buffer for the femoral condyles; fluid usually surrounds a tear
Symptoms	Trauma to knee, usually sports related Pain and swelling Difficulty in weight bearing and walking
Suggested protocols	Routine knee Best seen on sagittal and coronal images
Appearance	On T1 and T2, the menisci are black because they contain no hydrogen; tears in them appear as white inside the dark, triangular-shaped meniscus; a complete tear appears white all the way through the meniscus to the bony border of the knee; there is also fluid around most tears; fluid appears dark on T1 and white on T2 images
Contrast	None

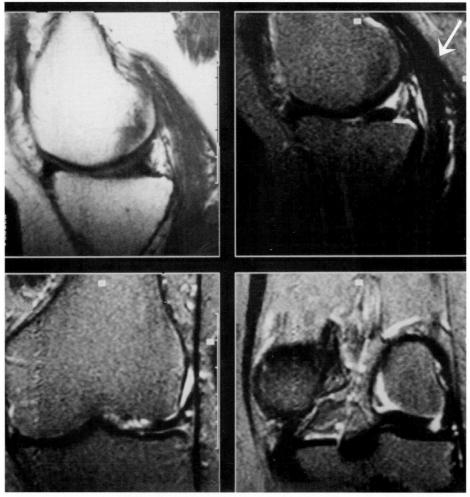

Figure 5-14 Medial meniscus tear, posterior horn
Upper left: proton density sagittal
Upper right: T2 sagittal
Lower left: T2 coronal
Lower right: T2 coronal

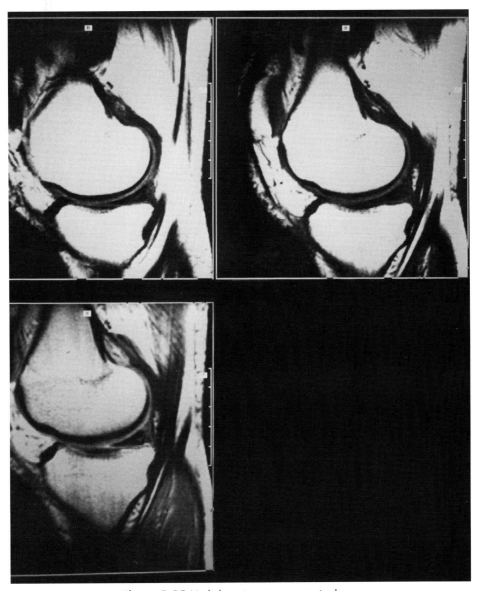

Figure 5–15 Medial meniscus tear, posterior horn
T1 sagittal

Chart 5–11. **Musculoskeletal** (Fig. 5–16)

Pathology	"Bucket handle" tear of medial meniscus
Description	Tear extends lengthwise from posterior to anterior horn; peripheral part of the meniscus is the "bucket," and the "handle" is the torn inner portion of the meniscus, which is displaced into the intercondylar notch
Symptoms	Twisting injury to the knee Locking of knee Pain and swelling
Suggested protocols	Routine knee
Appearance	Inner part of black meniscus displaced into intercondylar notch next to anterior cruciate ligament; irregular and narrowed outside margin of meniscus; tear appears white in black meniscus on all sequences
Contrast	None

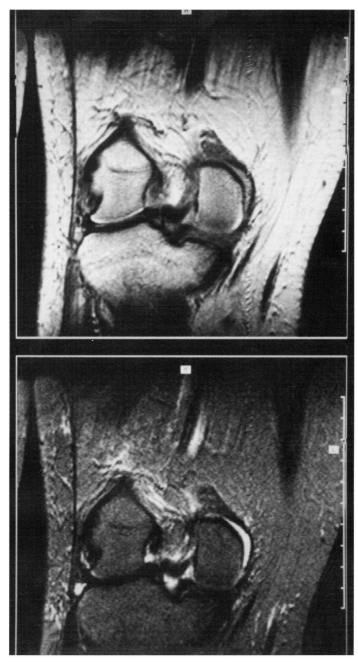

Figure 5-16 "Bucket handle" tear of medial meniscus
Upper: proton density coronal
Lower: T2 coronal

Chart 5–12. **Musculoskeletal** (Fig. 5–17)

Pathology	Anterior cruciate ligament tear
Description	Tear occurs more often at femoral insertion; usually accompanied by large hemarthrosis in joint space
Symptoms	An audible "pop" is heard at time of injury; an external force is placed on the knee or could be caused by sudden stopping or change of direction
Suggested protocols	Routine knee Possible 3-mm slices angled with anterior cruciate ligament if ligament not well seen on previous sequences
Appearance	Normally, the ligament is a black band crossing from the top of the joint space (femoral) to the bottom (tibial) on all imaging sequences; fluid around ligament appears white on T2 images and grayish on T1 because of blood and fluid mixture
Contrast	None

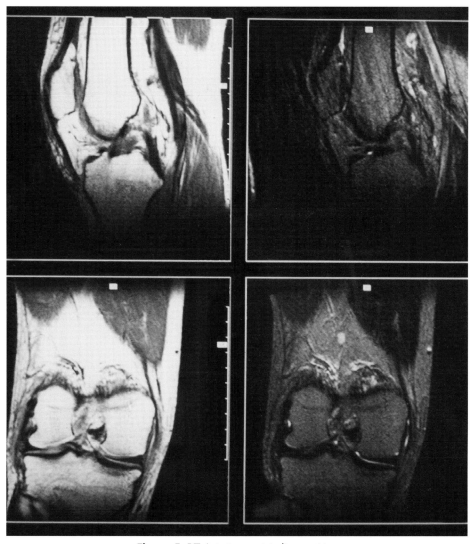

Figure 5-17 Anterior cruciate ligament tear
Upper left: T1 sagittal
Upper right: T2 sagittal
Lower left: proton density coronal
Lower right: T2 coronal

Chart 5–13. **Musculoskeletal** (Fig. 5–18)

Pathology	Lateral meniscal cyst in the knee
Description	Degenerative process of the meniscus can cause microcysts filled with synovial fluid; an intrameniscal cyst is within the margins of the meniscus but can grow outward with displacement of the joint capsule; usually on lateral menicus; these cysts generally do not become very large
Symptoms	Pain in knee Feeling of something "caught" in knee joint Asymptomatic until cyst becomes larger
Suggested protocols	Routine knee
Appearance	Well-defined area of white (fluid) on T2 images Well-defined area of dark (fluid) on T1 images
Contrast	None

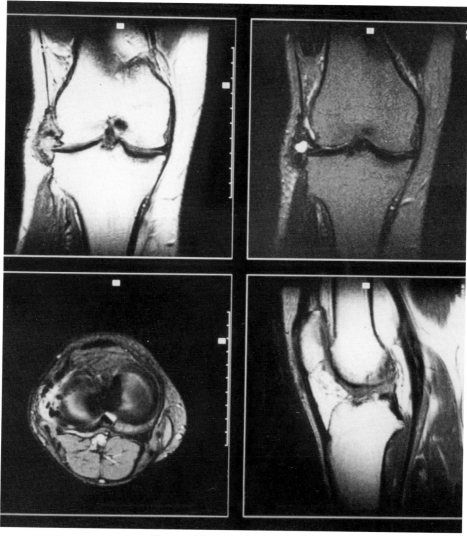

Figure 5–18 Lateral meniscal cyst
Upper left: proton density coronal
Upper right: T2 coronal
Lower left: gradient echo T2 axial
Lower right: T1 sagittal

Chart 5–14. **Musculoskeletal** (Figs. 5–19 and 5–20)

Pathology	Femur bone bruise
	Femur and tibia bone infarct
Description	Bone infarct: comes from lack of blood supply to area of bone marrow
	Bone bruise: trauma related, where there have been tiny fractures of the trabecular bone with hemorrhage and edema; involves the subchondral bone
Symptoms	Pain and swelling
	History of trauma to knee
Suggested protocols	Routine knee
Appearance	Infarct: dark edges in bone marrow surrounding infarct on T1, white edges surrounding infarct on T2 with grayish center
	Bruise: appears white on T2 and dark on T1
Contrast	To differentiate from other lesions

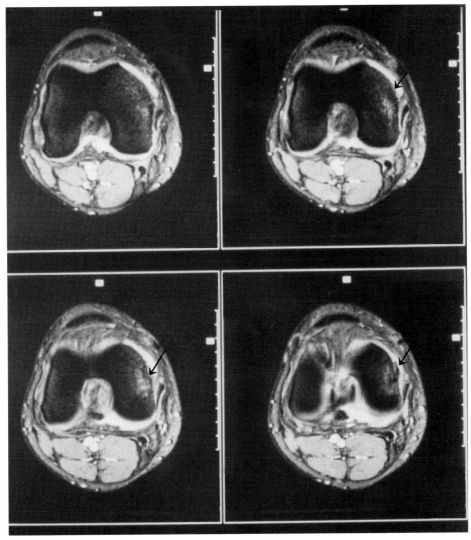

Figure 5-19 Bone bruise, femur
T2 axials

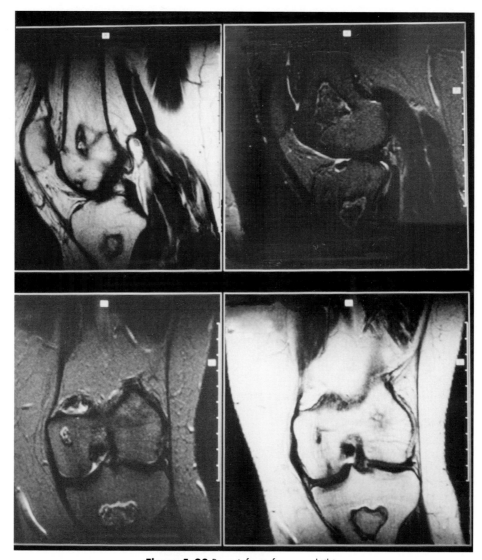

Figure 5-20 Bone infarct, femur and tibia
Upper left: T1 sagittal
Upper right: T2 sagittal
Lower left: T2 coronal
Lower right: T1 coronal

Chart 5–15. **Musculoskeletal** (Fig. 5–21)

Pathology	Bipartite patella
Description	Normal variant—failure of fusion of ossification centers
Symptoms	Incidental finding
Suggested protocols	Routine knee
Appearance	Patella appears as two pieces with dark edge separating them
Contrast	Dependent on radiologist

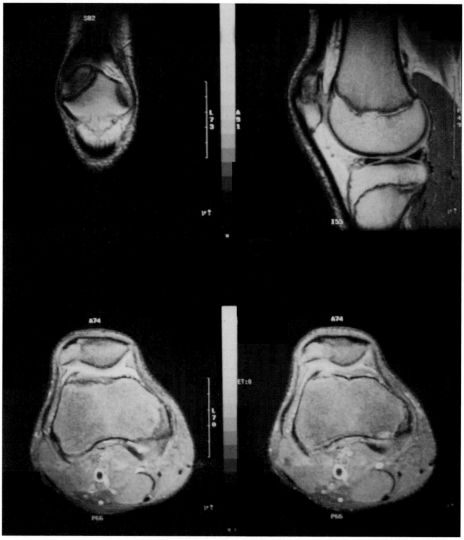

Figure 5-21 Bipartite patella
Upper left: T2 coronal
Upper right: T2 sagittal
Lower left: T2 axial
Lower right: T2 axial

Chart 5–16. **Musculoskeletal** (Fig. 5–22)

Pathology	Lesion of the tibia
Description	Differential includes chondroblastoma, which occurs in the epiphyseal region; may show some calcification; could be a simple cyst
Symptoms	Pain and swelling
Suggested protocols	Routine knee with larger FOV to obtain complete coverage of lesion
Appearance	T2 appearance is of mixed black and white, not well defined
Contrast	To visualize the lesion

FOV = field of view.

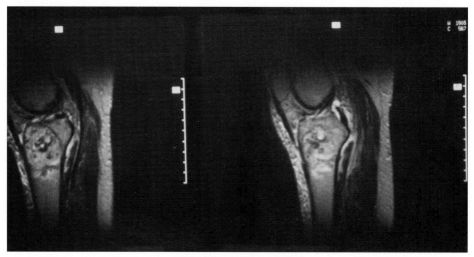

Figure 5–22 Lesion of tibia
T2 sagittals

Chart 5–17. **Musculoskeletal** (Fig. 5–23)

Pathology	Talus bone bruise
Description	Bone bruise is trauma related when there have been tiny fractures of the trabecular bone with hemorrhage and edema; involves subchondral bone
Symptoms	Pain and swelling with history of injury to foot
Suggested protocols	T1 sagittals and coronals T2 sagittals and coronals FOV = 240 mm Slice thickness = 4 mm
Appearance	T1 appears dark against lighter bone marrow T2 appears whiter against lighter bone marrow
Contrast	To differentiate from a lesion

FOV = field of view.

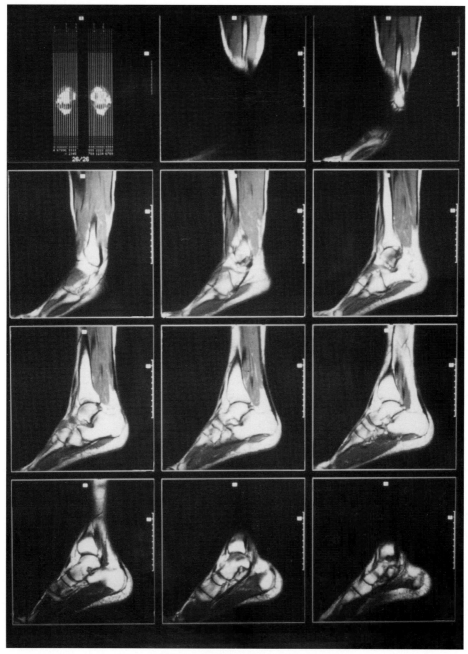

Figure 5–23 Talus bone bruise
T1 sagittals

Chart 5–18. **Musculoskeletal** (Figs. 5–24 and 5–25)

Pathology	First metatarsal lesion (big toe) Possible pathologic fracture
Description	Differential diagnosis of such a toe lesion could include an osteoid osteoma, which is a benign lesion located in the cortex of bone or cancellous bone; a second differential might be an "osteochondroma," which is a benign lesion in the bone marrow, occurring in children and adolescents
Symptoms	Pain and swelling from fracture Asymptomatic
Suggested protocols	T1 axials, coronals, and sagittals T2 axials, coronals, and sagittals FOV = 150 mm Slice thickness = 3–4 mm Matrix = 256 × 256
Appearance	Lesion appears dark grayish in the whiter bone marrow on T1 and whitish in the gray bone marrow on T2
Contrast	To enhance lesion and invasion into soft tissue

FOV = field of view.

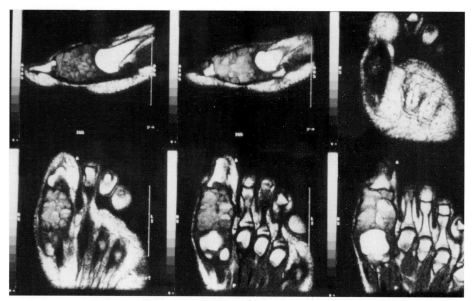

Figure 5–24 First metatarsal lesion with pathologic fracture
Upper left: T1 sagittal
Upper middle: T1 sagittal
Upper right: T1 coronal
Lower: T1 coronal

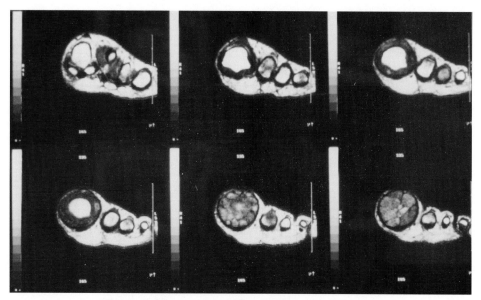

Figure 5–25 First metatarsal lesion with pathologic fracture
T1 axials

CHAPTER SIX

Summary

It is hoped that this pathology atlas allows the reader to delve into disease processes with more vigor. It has perhaps provided a solid background and additional tools to research, scan, and study other disease processes in one's own environment (Fig. 6–1). I encourage all readers to put themselves in the place of the patient in dealing with endless testing involved in the diagnosis of a serious illness. Knowing more about the diseases will make this easier.

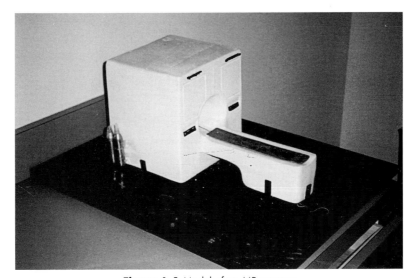

Figure 6–1 Model of an MR scanner.

Bibliography

Applegate E. The sectional anatomy learning system. Philadelphia: WB Saunders, 1991.

Barrett C, Anderson L, Holder L. Primer of sectional anatomy with MRI and CT correlation. Baltimore, MD: Williams & Wilkins, 1994.

Barrett C, Poliakoff S, Holder L. Primer of sectional anatomy with MRI and CT correlation. Baltimore, MD: Williams & Wilkins, 1994.

Chandrasoma P, Taylor CR. Concise pathology, 2nd ed. Norwalk, CT: Appleton & Lange, 1995.

Firooznia H, Golimbu C, Rafil M. MRI and CT of the musculoskeletal system. St. Louis, MO: Mosby–Year Book, 1991.

Latchaw R. MR and CT imaging of the head, neck, and spine, 2nd ed. St. Louis, MO: Mosby–Year Book, 1991.

Mulvihill MLou. Human diseases—a systemic approach. Norwalk, CT: Appleton & Lange, 1995.

Robbins S, Cotran R, Kumar V. Pocket companion to Robbins pathologic basis of disease. Philadelphia: WB Saunders, 1991.

Index

ISBN 0-7216-6416-4

90038

9 780721 664163